FIFTH EDITION

WORKBOOK FOR
JOHNS HOPKINS EVIDENCE-BASED PRACTICE
FOR NURSES AND HEALTHCARE PROFESSIONALS

Model & Guidelines

Kim Bissett, PhD, MBA, RN
Alexandra Johnson, MPH, MSN, RN

Copyright © 2025 by Sigma Theta Tau International Honor Society of Nursing

All rights reserved. This book is protected by copyright. No part of it may be reproduced, stored in a retrieval system, or transmitted in any form or by any means, electronic, mechanical, photocopying, recording, or otherwise, without written permission from the publisher. Any trademarks, service marks, design rights, or similar rights that are mentioned, used, or cited in this book are the property of their respective owners. Their use here does not imply that you may use them for a similar or any other purpose.

This book is not intended to be a substitute for the medical advice of a licensed medical professional. The author and publisher have made every effort to ensure the accuracy of the information contained within at the time of its publication and shall have no liability or responsibility to any person or entity regarding any loss or damage incurred, or alleged to have incurred, directly or indirectly, by the information contained in this book. The author and publisher make no warranties, express or implied, with respect to its content, and no warranties may be created or extended by sales representatives or written sales materials. The author and publisher have no responsibility for the consistency or accuracy of URLs and content of third-party websites referenced in this book.

> *Sigma Theta Tau International Honor Society of Nursing (Sigma) is a nonprofit organization whose mission is developing nurse leaders anywhere to improve healthcare everywhere. Founded in 1922, Sigma has more than 80,000 active members in over 100 countries and territories. Members include practicing nurses, instructors, researchers, policymakers, entrepreneurs, and others. Sigma's 600 chapters are located at more than 700 institutions of higher education throughout Armenia, Australia, Botswana, Brazil, Canada, Chile, Colombia, Croatia, England, Eswatini, Finland, Ghana, Hong Kong, Ireland, Israel, Italy, Jamaica, Japan, Jordan, Kenya, Lebanon, Malawi, Mexico, the Netherlands, Nigeria, Pakistan, Philippines, Portugal, Puerto Rico, Saudi Arabia, Scotland, Singapore, South Africa, South Korea, Spain, Sweden, Taiwan, Tanzania, Thailand, the United States, and Wales. Learn more at www.sigmanursing.org.*

Sigma Theta Tau International
550 West North Street
Indianapolis, IN, USA 46202

To request a review copy for course adoption, order additional books, buy in bulk, or purchase for corporate use, contact Sigma Marketplace at 888.654.4968 (US/Canada toll-free), +1.317.687.2256 (International), or solutions@sigmamarketplace.org.

To request author information, or for speaker or other media requests, contact Sigma Marketing at 888.634.7575 (US/Canada toll-free) or +1.317.634.8171 (International).

ISBN: 9781646481385
PDF ISBN: 9781646481392

Publisher: Dustin Sullivan
Acquisitions Editor: Emily Hatch
Development Editor: Jillmarie Leeper Sycamore
Cover Designer: Rebecca Batchelor
Interior Design/Page Layout: Rebecca Batchelor

Managing Editor: Carla Hall
Publications Specialist: Todd Lothery
Project Editor: Todd Lothery
Copy Editor: Todd Lothery
Proofreader: Todd Lothery

DEDICATION

This workbook is dedicated to all those on the journey of lifelong learning.
May you never stop inquiring, exploring, and seeking to understand.

ACKNOWLEDGMENTS

We would like to acknowledge the Johns Hopkins Center for Nursing Inquiry for the tremendous work they have done to disseminate evidence-based practice information via podcasts, many of which we have selected for this workbook.

ABOUT THE AUTHORS

Kim Bissett, PhD, MBA, RN, is a nurse educator and Director of EBP at the Institute for Johns Hopkins Nursing. She has been involved with the Johns Hopkins Evidence-Based Practice (JHEBP) model for many years including as an EBP Fellow, a hospital-based EBP Coordinator, and a workshop facilitator. She has extensive experience in EBP education, presenting and consulting on evidence-based nursing practice nationally and internationally. Bissett assisted with developing and publishing previous editions of the *Johns Hopkins Nursing Evidence-Based Practice: Model and Guidelines.* She also teaches part time in the Johns Hopkins University School of Nursing's Doctor of Nursing Practice Program. Her research interests include self-compassion and fostering nurse well-being.

Alexandra Johnson, MPH, MSN, RN, is a Program Coordinator for the Department of Nursing at the Johns Hopkins Hospital. In this role, she conducts and guides nursing research, evidence-based practice, and quality improvement work. Originally from Chicago, Johnson relocated to Maryland in 2018 to join the Johns Hopkins Hospital as a nurse in the neonatal intensive care unit, where she continues to work clinically part time. Johnson is also adjunct faculty at the Johns Hopkins University School of Nursing.

CONTRIBUTING AUTHORS

Judith Ascenzi, DNP, RN, is the Director of Pediatric Nursing Programs for Education, Informatics, and Research at the Johns Hopkins Children's Center. She also teaches part time in the Johns Hopkins University School of Nursing's Doctorate of Nursing Practice Program. Ascenzi has presented and consulted nationally on the topic of evidence-based practice. She has served as expert facilitator on many evidence-based practice projects in her pediatric practice setting as well as with her adult colleagues at the Johns Hopkins Hospital. Ascenzi acts as a project advisor and organizational mentor for many doctoral students utilizing the JHEBP model as the foundational model for their projects.

Brenda Douglass, DNP, APRN, FNP-C, CDCES, CNE, CTTS, is a family nurse practitioner, Assistant Professor, and Associate Director of the DNP-AP Program – Project Focus at the Johns Hopkins University School of Nursing. She brings a wealth of experience and leadership, integrating academic, clinical, research, and leadership roles throughout her career. A recognized leader in nursing education, she provides program oversight of DNP projects, project core courses, and practicum experiences, ensuring alignment with accreditation standards, competency-based education, and evidence-based practice. Douglass is actively involved in advancing DNP education through initiatives focused on enhancing project and practicum experiences, integrating competency-based education and strengthening academic-practice partnerships. Douglass serves on national and university committees focused on nursing education, leadership, and policy and is a dedicated mentor and advisor committed to developing future nurse leaders and educators who are prepared to drive healthcare transformation through evidence-based practice and quality improvement initiatives.

Lisa Grubb, DNP, MSN, BSN, RN, CWCN, CPHQ, C/DONA, is an Assistant Professor at the Johns Hopkins University School of Nursing, where she coordinates and teaches in the DNP/AP project courses. She uses the Johns Hopkins Evidence-Based Practice model as a foundation for all DNP project courses. Before her current role, she was the Senior Director of Quality and Patient Safety at the Johns Hopkins Howard County Medical Center, where she focused on using evidence-based practices to improve patient outcomes, including reducing length of stay, decreasing readmissions, and enhancing patient satisfaction and value-based care. Additionally, she has collaborated with the Institute for Johns Hopkins Nursing and the Johns Hopkins Nursing Administration to support nurses in evidence-based practice, knowledge translation, and quality improvement research projects. Grubb has a strong interest in promoting EBP in both clinical settings and academic environments.

Madeleine Whalen, MSN/MPH, RN, CEN, NPD-BC, is the Evidence-Based Practice Program Coordinator for the Johns Hopkins Health System. In this role she educates and supports frontline nurses in completing robust and actionable EBP projects rooted in bedside experience. She began her nursing career in the emergency department while earning her master's degrees in nursing and public health. She is a Joanna Briggs Institute Scientific Writer and a member of the *Journal of Emergency Nursing* editorial board. She continues to work clinically part time and serves as adjunct faculty at the Johns Hopkins University School of Nursing and the Johns Hopkins Medicine Center for Global Emergency Care. Her professional interests include global health, evidence synthesis, and empowering nurses to advance the profession and science of nursing through inquiry.

TABLE OF CONTENTS

About the Authors v
Contributing Authors vi
Introduction ix

1 Evidence-Based Practice: Past, Present, and Future 2

2 The Johns Hopkins Evidence-Based Practice (JHEBP) Model for Nurses and Healthcare Professionals (HCPs) Process Overview 8

3 Practice Question Phase: The Problem 18

4 Practice Question Phase: The EBP Question 26

5 The Interprofessional Team 36

6 Evidence Phase: Introduction to Evidence 42

7 Evidence Phase: The Evidence Search and Screening 50

8 Evidence Phase: Appraising the Evidence 62

9 Evidence Phase: Summary, Synthesis, and Best-Evidence Recommendations 84

10 Translation Phase: Translation 96

11 Translation Phase: Implementation 102

12 Ongoing Considerations: Communication and Dissemination 108

INTRODUCTION TO THE WORKBOOK

This workbook complements *Johns Hopkins Evidence-Based Practice for Nurses and Healthcare Professionals: Model & Guidelines*, Fifth Edition. This workbook offers additional resources and learning activities to deepen understanding of the content and provide additional perspectives. It may be used as an ancillary to coursework in a classroom or independently for self-guided learning.

The workbook is divided into chapters mirroring the text. Each workbook chapter provides:

- A chapter overview
- A list of key points
- Learning objectives
- Links to associated resources
- Activities to enhance learning
- Call to Action segments that direct users to complete steps in the evidence-based practice (EBP) process for teams working on actual EBP projects
- Discussion questions
- A closer look at annotated tools where applicable

Some of the exercises in the workbook are based on one fictitious clinical scenario.

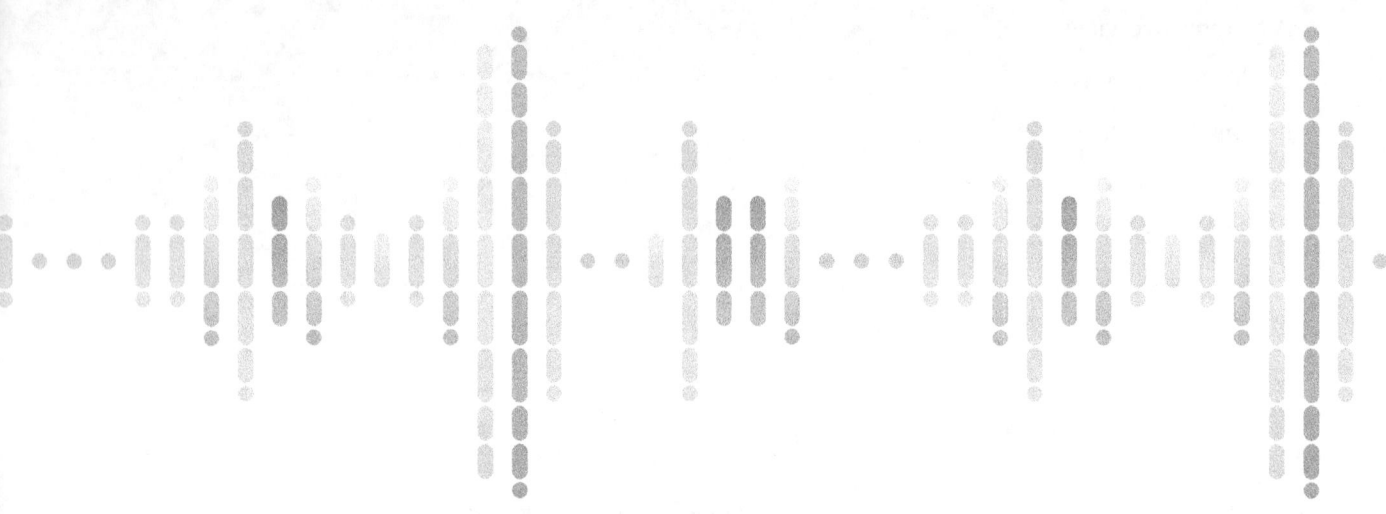

OVERVIEW

This chapter defines *evidence-based practice* (EBP) and discusses the evolution that led to the focus on using evidence-based practices to guide decision-making. EBP creates a culture of critical thinking and ongoing learning and is the foundation for an environment where evidence supports clinical, operational, and educational decisions. EBP is an explicit process that facilitates decision-making to support effective, efficient, and equitable patient-centered care.

Recent global challenges such as COVID-19 highlighted the need for clinicians to be well-versed in rapidly accessing and appraising available evidence for practice or adapting in the absence of evidence. Despite many advances in EBP and access to evidence, healthcare professionals continue to practice by tradition, and barriers to EBP still exist. Emerging technologies such as artificial intelligence (AI) promise to make EBP more accessible or replace it altogether. However, even those advances would still require clinicians knowledgeable in the EBP process to verify AI findings. Healthcare equality can be addressed through EBP and should be a regular consideration starting at the local level.

EVIDENCE-BASED PRACTICE: PAST, PRESENT, AND FUTURE

KEY POINTS

- EBP helps clinicians keep up with emerging evidence, practices, and technologies.

- The Johns Hopkins Evidence-Based Practice (JHEBP) Model for Nursing and Healthcare Professionals provides a structured and systematic way for clinicians to effectively use current scientific and experiential evidence to determine best practices and provide safe, high-quality care.

- Numerous healthcare organizations encourage the use and prioritization of EBP.

- EBP can be used during resource-limited times such as with the COVID-19 pandemic. Clinicians may need to think creatively and expand their skill sets.

- AI can potentially enhance the EBP process by speeding up the process or replacing many of the human tasks. In the future, AI may complete entire EBP projects in seconds.

- EBP teams can address health equity locally by considering diversity, equity, and inclusion from the start of the EBP project.

OBJECTIVES

- 1.1 Compare and contrast practice based on evidence and one based on tradition (analyzing)

- 1.2 Describe three ways AI may promote EBP (understanding)

- 1.3 Demonstrate how EBP can be used to address health equity on a local level (applying)

LEARNING ACTIVITIES

Before completion of the learning activities, you should do the following:

- Read Chapter 1
- Read the article at https://nursingaura.com/44-difference-between-evidence-based-practice-and-traditional-nursing/

Learning Activity 1.1

Create a table differentiating evidence-based and tradition-based practices.

CHARACTERISTICS	EBP	TRADITION
Definition		
Foundation		
Process		
Flexibility		
Outcome orientation		
Evaluation		

Learning Activity 1.2

Identify and describe three ways AI may promote EBP.

_____

_____

_____

_____

Learning Activity 1.3

Read the following case study excerpt, and, in the space that follows, outline the steps the team should take or consider to address health equity through the EBP process.

You work as a nurse in an adult medical/surgical unit at a small community hospital. On December 1st, Ms. J, a 68-year-old Black woman, was admitted to your unit from the emergency department for pneumonia. She had a peripheral intravenous (IV) catheter in place and was receiving IV antibiotics. She was also receiving supplemental oxygen via a nasal cannula and nebulizer treatments every four hours. Ms. J did not have any other medical conditions and was not taking any other medications.

That day, you were working the night shift, 1900 to 0700, and assigned to care for Ms. J. You received in report that Ms. J did not have a history of falls, did not require any ambulatory aids, and used her call bell for assistance. At the start of your shift, Ms. J was seated in a chair chatting with visitors. You completed your fall risk assessment using a scored screening tool, which determined that Ms. J was a low risk for falls. You also completed an environmental safety check; you did not observe any slip, trip, or fall hazards at that time. As you left the room, you instructed Ms. J to ring her call bell if she needed any assistance.

The next couple hours of your shift were busy. A new patient was admitted to your hallway from surgery. Even though you were not assigned to admit the patient, you were the most experienced nurse in your hallway and were needed as a resource.

At 2330, you heard Ms. J shouting for help from the hallway. You found Ms. J on the floor; she tripped and fell on her way to the bathroom. As you entered the room to help, you noticed multiple new environmental hazards. Since you last performed your environmental safety check, someone had added extension tubing to Ms. J's nasal cannula, and the extra tubing was tangled around her IV pole. Her visitors had also left, and there were chairs scattered about the room.

As a result of her fall, Ms. J broke her hip, which will require surgery. This will increase her hospital stay, increase her healthcare costs, and decrease her quality of life.

During your root cause analysis, you discover that Ms. J's fall is not an isolated incident. Over the past quarter, there has been a 35% increase in falls on your unit. The falls on your unit were caused by a variety of issues but most commonly occurred because of patient-related factors (e.g., age, medical conditions, medications, etc.) or environmental factors (e.g., clutter, wet floors, poor lighting, etc.).

_____

_____

_____

_____

_____

CALL TO ACTION

Consider your own work. Are there practices based on tradition rather than evidence? Are there opportunities to improve using EBP? This may be a good place to start if you are looking for a topic for an EBP project.

DISCUSSION QUESTIONS

1. What are the primary barriers to implementing EBP in clinical settings, and how might healthcare organizations work to overcome these obstacles?

2. How did the COVID-19 pandemic underscore the importance of EBP for clinicians, particularly in terms of quickly accessing and evaluating available evidence? What lessons can be learned for future healthcare challenges?

3. In what ways could emerging technologies, like AI, change the landscape of EBP? What role should clinicians play in ensuring the reliability and accuracy of AI-generated evidence?

4. How can EBP be leveraged to address healthcare inequalities? What strategies could be implemented to ensure that EBP considerations start at the local level and address diverse community needs?

5. Despite advancements in EBP, some healthcare providers continue to rely on traditional practices. What factors contribute to this reliance, and how can a culture of critical thinking and continuous learning be fostered to encourage wider adoption of EBP?

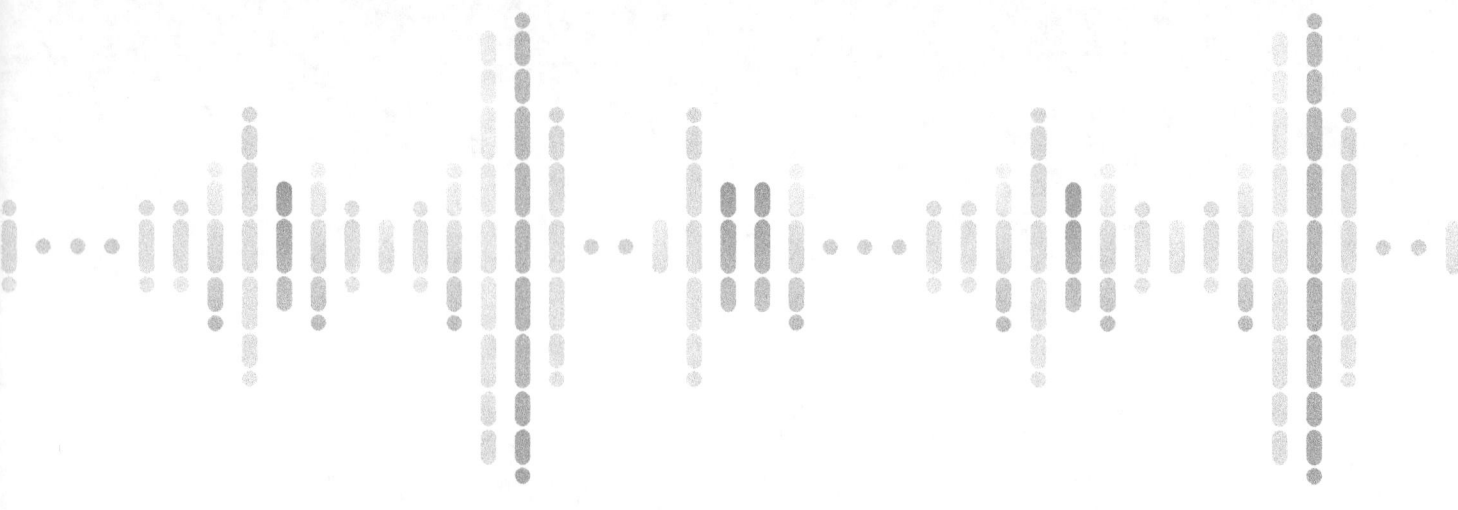

OVERVIEW

EBP is a core competency for all healthcare professionals (HCPs) in all practice settings (Saunders et al., 2019). Using an evidence-based approach to care and practice decision-making is not only an expectation in all practice settings but also a requirement established by professional standards, regulatory agencies, health insurers, and purchasers of healthcare insurance. EBP is an important component of high-reliability organizations. It is a process that can enable organizations to meet the quadruple healthcare aim to enhance patient care, improve population health, reduce healthcare costs, and increase the well-being of healthcare staff (Migliore et al., 2020).

This chapter introduces the revised JHEBP model (2024) and the 16 steps of the PET process, designed as an intentional and systematic approach to EBP that requires support and commitment at the individual, team, and organizational levels. HCPs with varied experience and educational preparation have successfully used this process with coaching, mentorship, and organizational support (Dearholt & Dang, 2012).

2

THE JOHNS HOPKINS EVIDENCE-BASED PRACTICE (JHEBP) MODEL FOR NURSES AND HEALTHCARE PROFESSIONALS (HCPs) PROCESS OVERVIEW

KEY POINTS

This chapter summarizes all the steps in the JHEBP model. The EBP Project Steps and Overview (Appendix A) mirrors this overview.

- Quality improvement (QI), research, and EBP are the three forms of inquiry common to healthcare.

- The JHEBP model is built on the concepts of inquiry, practice, and learning.

- Critical thinking and clinical reasoning are essential components of the model.

- The EBP process can be influenced by both internal and external factors.

- The JHEBP model uses the PET process: Practice Question, Evidence, and Translation.

- The JHEBP model consists of 16 steps with associated tools to guide the EBP process.

OBJECTIVES

- 2.1 Differentiate between QI, EBP, and research (analyzing)

- 2.2 Describe the JHEBP model and PET process (understanding)

- 2.3 Demonstrate knowledge of the appropriate steps in the PET process (applying)

LEARNING ACTIVITIES

Before completion of the learning activities, you should do the following:

- Read Chapter 2
- Listen to the podcast at https://podcasts.apple.com/us/podcast/ep-4-johns-hopkins-nursing-center-for-nursing-inquiry/id1478145611?i=1000448670863
- Download the EBP Project Steps and Overview (Appendix A; Hopkins.org/tools) and the Gantt chart (Hopkins.org/resources)

Learning Activity 2.1

Part 1: In your own words, define the following:

Quality improvement	
Research	
Evidence-based practice	

Part 2: Given the following statements, select the appropriate category (QI, research, or EBP).

_____ The nurses in Labor and Delivery at XYZ Hospital want to improve the time it takes for new mothers to be evaluated by the lactation nurse.

_____ A group from ABC University wants to better understand the impact of social media on children born to single parents.

_____ The Nursing Department at XYZ Hospital wants to ensure they provide the best support for families of children recently diagnosed with leukemia.

Learning Activity 2.2

Describe what sparks an EBP project. Once initiated, what are the three phases the team will move through? What happens in each of those phases?

___

___

___

___

___

Learning Activity 2.3

Order the 16 steps of the JHEBP model by placing the correct numbers in front of each step.

_____ Create an implementation/action plan

_____ Write the EBP question

_____ Assess the risk, fit, feasibility, and acceptability of best-evidence recommendations

_____ Summarize the evidence

_____ Conduct targeted search or exhaustive search and screening

_____ Conduct best-evidence search and appraisal

_____ Record best-evidence recommendations

_____ Identify practice-setting specific recommendations

_____ Organize the data

_____ Implement

_____ Explore and describe the problem

_____ Monitor sustainability and identify next steps

_____ Appraise the evidence

_____ Synthesize the findings

_____ Identify an implementation framework

_____ Develop the problem statement

CALL TO ACTION

The EBP Project Steps and Overview (Appendix A; see Figures 2.1 and 2.2) provides a snapshot of the steps in the EBP process. Once your team has identified the problem and EBP question, return to page 2 of the Project Steps and Overview and use the decision tree to determine 1) if EBP is the appropriate approach and 2) the type of search required for your question.

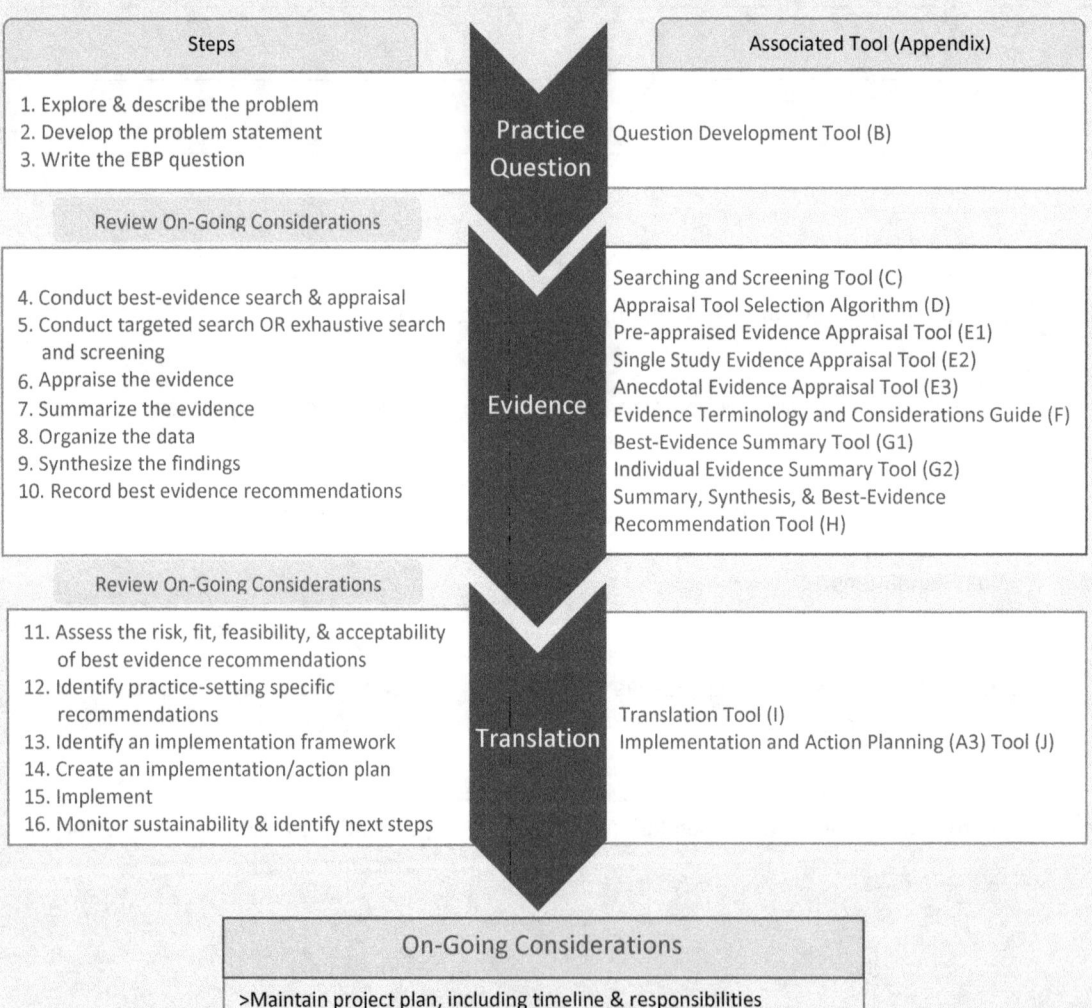

FIGURE 2.1 EBP Project Steps and Overview (Appendix A), front side.

Evidence Phase Decision Tree:

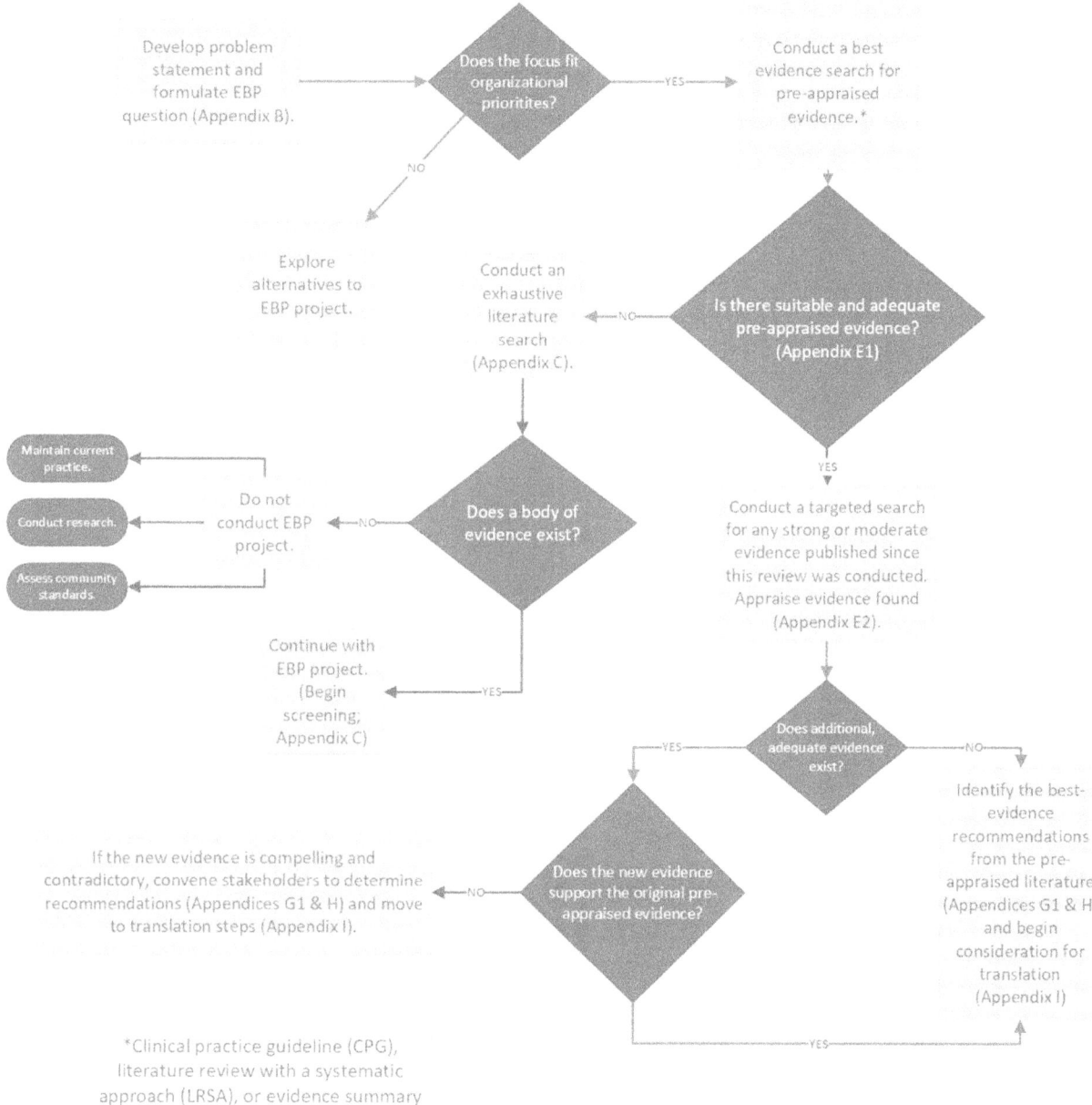

FIGURE 2.2 EBP Project Steps and Overview (Appendix A), back side.

DISCUSSION QUESTIONS

1. What are the key components of the revised JHEBP model, and how does this updated framework improve upon previous versions in supporting effective EBP?
2. The PET process consists of 16 steps. How can healthcare organizations ensure that healthcare professionals are adequately trained and supported at each step of the process to successfully implement EBP?
3. How can coaching and mentorship contribute to the success of EBP initiatives? What strategies could be employed to foster these relationships within healthcare teams?
4. What role does organizational commitment play in the successful adoption of the PET process? How can leaders at various levels promote a culture that values EBP?
5. Healthcare professionals come from diverse educational backgrounds and levels of experience. What are some ways that organizations can tailor EBP training to accommodate this diversity, ensuring that all staff are equipped to utilize the PET process effectively?

A CLOSER LOOK

The EBP Project Steps and Overview (Appendix A)

This appendix outlines the steps in the PET process (see Figure 2.3) and factors the team should consider throughout the project. The tools and guides available for the project are listed according to the process phase. Additionally, the decision tree guides teams in determining if an EBP project is the correct path and what kind of search is required.

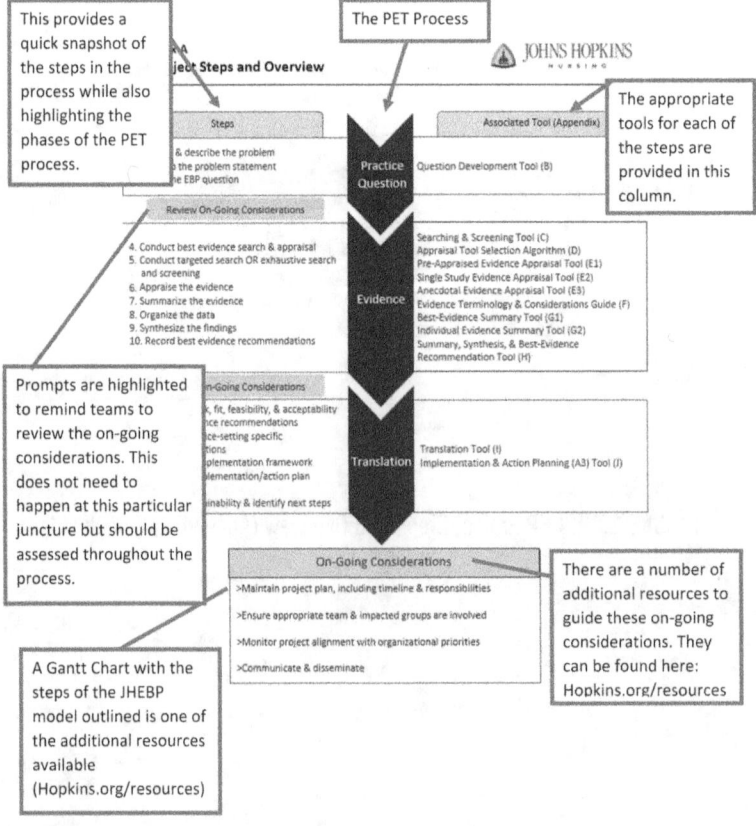

FIGURE 2.3 Annotation of the EBP Project Steps and Overview, Appendix A, front side.

THE GANTT CHART

EBP teams can track progress using many methods. One of the easiest is the Gantt chart (see Figure 2.4). It allows teams to plan out the project, celebrate reaching milestones, and recognize areas that may be lagging. A modifiable Gantt chart specific to the steps of the JHEBP model can be found here: Hopkins.org/resources.

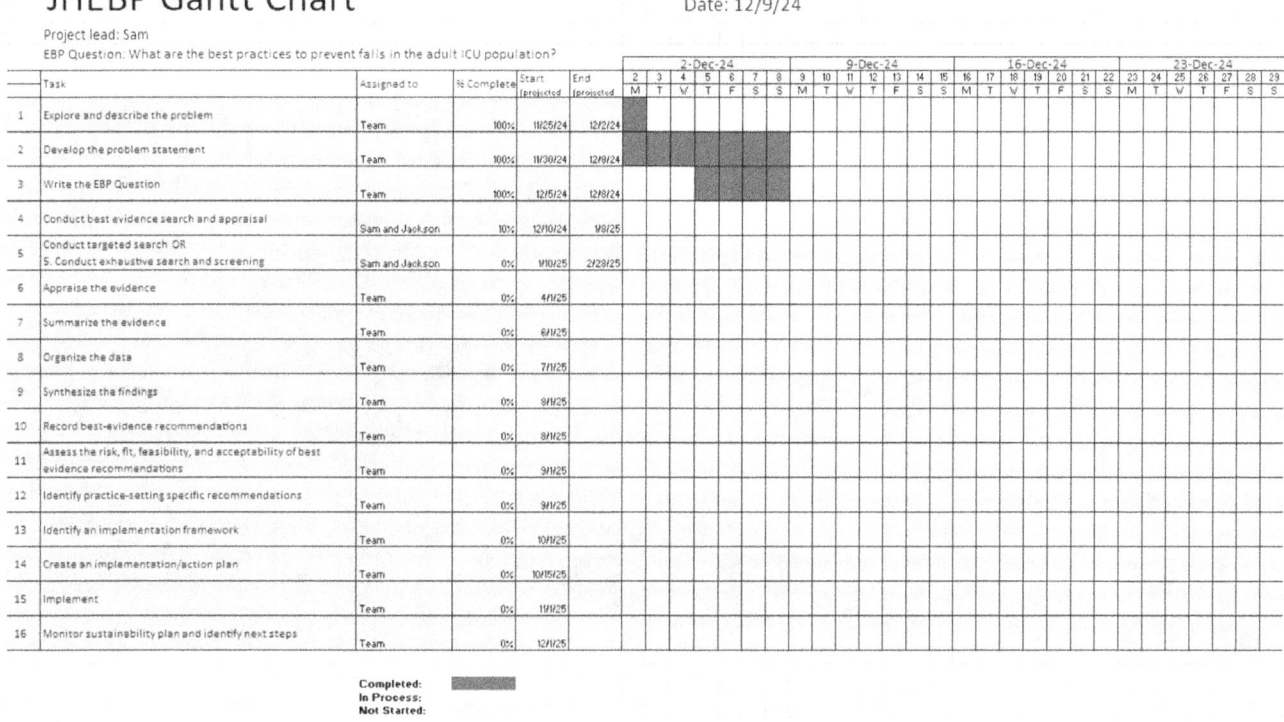

FIGURE 2.4   Gantt chart.

Using the decision tree (see Figure 2.5) in the EBP Project Steps and Overview (Appendix A) allows teams to determine 1) if an EBP project is the correct path and 2) what type of search is necessary for the given EBP question.

An EBP project may not be the best course of action if the focus does not meet organizational priorities or if sufficient evidence cannot be found. The decision tree also prompts teams to start with a targeted search. Prioritizing pre-appraised evidence saves time and energy, potentially allowing teams to move right into implementation.

Evidence Phase Decision Tree:

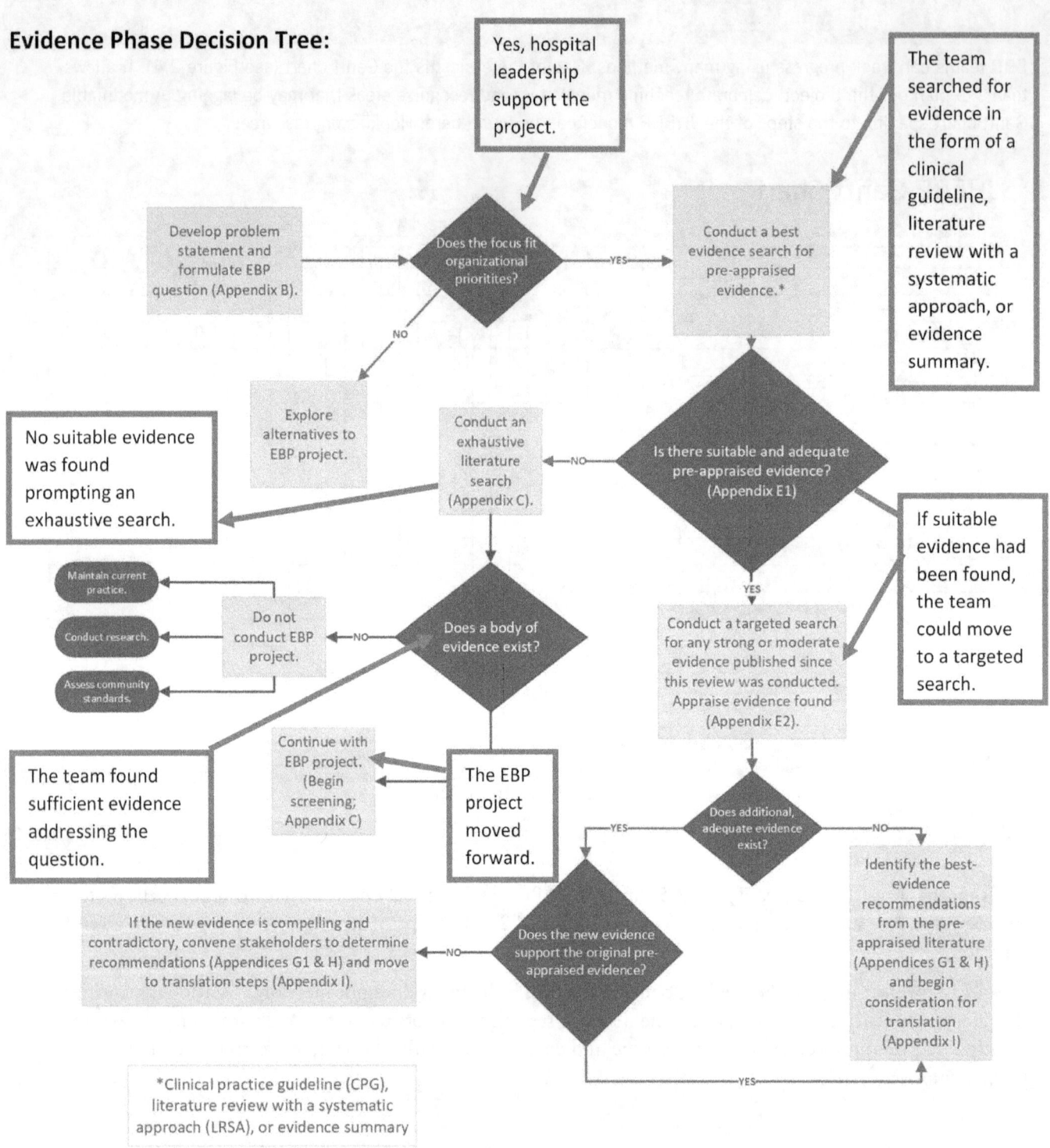

FIGURE 2.5 Evidence phase decision tree (Appendix A, back side), annotated.

REFERENCES

Dearholt, S. L., & Dang, D. (2012). *Johns Hopkins nursing evidence-based practice: Model and guidelines* (2nd ed.). Sigma Theta Tau International.

Migliore, L., Chouinard, H., & Woodlee, R. (2020). Clinical research and practice collaborative: An evidence-based nursing clinical inquiry expansion. *Military Medicine, 185*(2), 35–42. https://doi.org/10.1093/milmed/usz447

Saunders, H., Gallagher-Ford, L., Kvist, T., & Vehvilainen-Julkunen, K. (2019). Practicing HCPs' evidence-based practice competencies: An overview of systematic reviews. *Worldviews on Evidence-Based Nursing, 16*(3), 176–185. https://doi.org/10.1111/wvn.12363

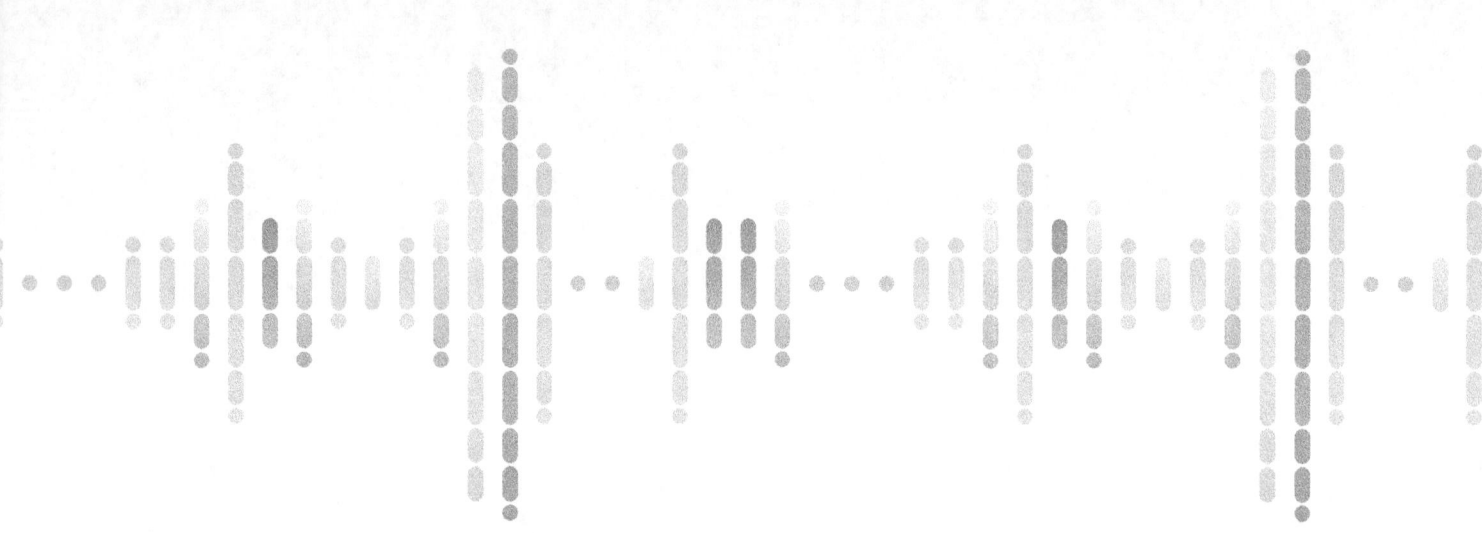

OVERVIEW

The practice question phase is the first phase of the PET process. EBP projects are born out of questions, curiosities, problems, or other issues that require further investigation. Exploring and establishing the problem lays the foundation for the project's trajectory and ensures efforts are focused on addressing not only the correct problem but also problems that are well-suited to the EBP process.

3

PRACTICE QUESTION PHASE: THE PROBLEM

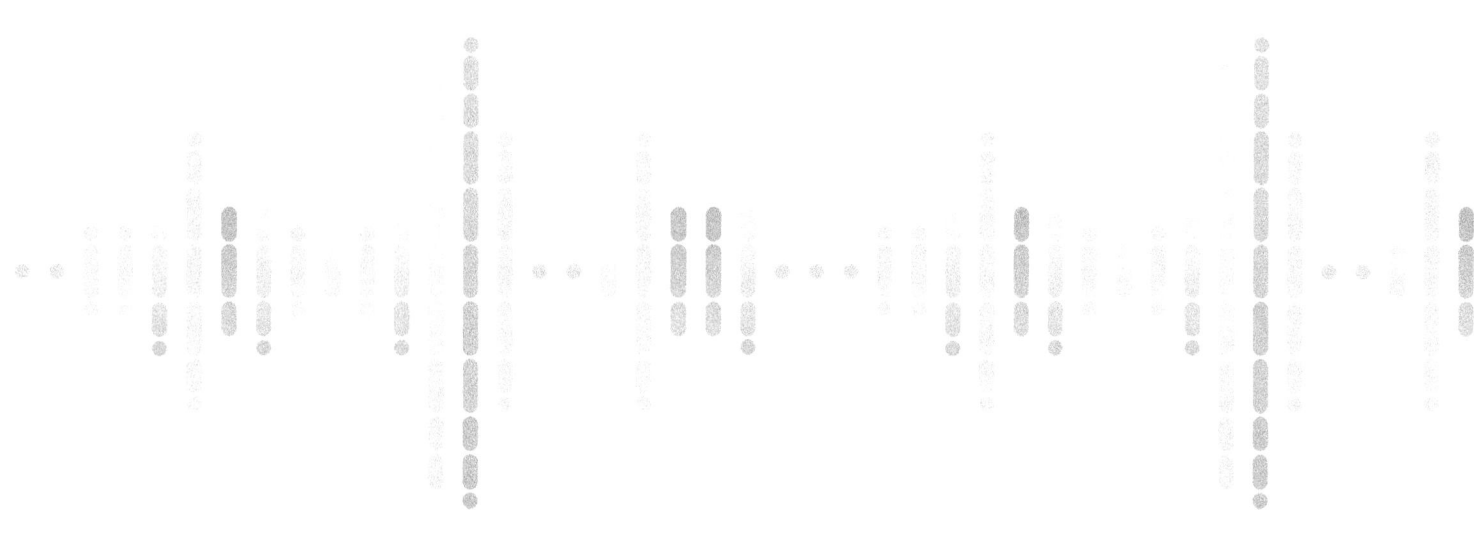

KEY POINTS

The practice question phase contains three steps. This chapter reviews the first and second steps. The JHEBP Question Development Tool (Appendix B) facilitates this phase.

- Failing to fully describe and define the problem can lead to ineffective solutions.

- Teams should avoid starting with a solution in mind, focusing on the symptoms of the problem, and jumping on the first problem identified.

- Spending time exploring the problem with techniques such as a root cause analysis will help identify the true problem.

- Inaccurate or poorly defined problem statements may lead to wasted time, resources, and potential dead ends in the EBP process.

OBJECTIVES

- 3.1 Identify strategies used to define problems (understanding)

- 3.2 Differentiate between problems, solutions, and symptoms (analyzing)

- 3.3 Construct a problem statement (creating)

LEARNING ACTIVITIES

Before completion of the learning activities, you should do the following:

- Read Chapter 3
- Read this article: https://online.hbs.edu/blog/post/root-cause-analysis
- Review the Question Development Tool (Appendix B)
- Download the Fishbone diagram from the resources page (Hopkins.org/resources)

Learning Activity 3.1

Draw a line to match each strategy with the corresponding rationale.

STRATEGY	RATIONALE
Examine the problem critically without making assumptions to ensure that the final statement defines the specific problem.	Helps gain clarity by using different verbs
Challenge assumptions.	Allows the team to assess the current state and envision a future state in which broken components are fixed, risks are prevented, new evidence is accepted, and missing elements are provided
Ask clarifying questions.	Helps the team understand whether the problem is part of a larger problem or is made up of many smaller problems
State the problem differently.	Keeps the team focused on processes and systems as the team moves to define the EBP question
Expand and contract the problem.	Helps the team get to the specific problem by using question words such as when, what, and how
Refrain from blaming the problem on external forces or focusing attention on the wrong aspect of the problem.	Gives the team time to gather information, observe, listen, and probe to ensure a true understanding of the problem
Describe in precise terms the perceived gap between what one sees and what one wants to see.	Helps the team avoid conjecture and question everyday processes and practices that are taken for granted

Learning Activity 3.2

Identify whether the following statements describe the symptom(s) of a problem, a problem, or a solution to a problem.

1. Central venous catheters (CVC) are necessary tools to care for critically ill patients. However, improper insertion, maintenance, and removal of central lines can lead to bacterial and fungal infections.

    a. Symptoms of a problem

    b. Problem

    c. Solution to a problem

2. There is an increase in central line–associated bloodstream infections (CLABSIs) in the Department of Surgery at a large, academic medical center. CLABSIs can lead to increased length of stay, healthcare costs, and morbidity and mortality.

    a. Symptoms of a problem

    b. Problem

    c. Solution to a problem

3. Using an equipment bundle when inserting a central line can help reduce CLABSIs. A central line equipment bundle includes and organizes all the equipment needed to prepare, insert, secure, and dress a CVC.

    a. Symptoms of a problem

    b. Problem

    c. Solution to a problem

Learning Activity 3.3

Complete the problems portion of the Question Development Tool (see Figure 3.1) using the case study excerpt from Chapter 1 of this workbook.

Question Development Tool

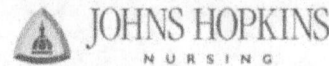

> Purpose: This form guides the EBP team in developing an answerable EBP question. It is meant to be fluid and dynamic as the team engages in the question development process. As the team becomes familiar with the evidence base for the topic of interest, they revisit, revise, and refine the question, search terms, search strategy, and sources of evidence.

*If viewing this online, hover over bold text for more information

What is the local problem? *(the response can be a bulleted list or phrases)*

Why is this problem important and relevant? What would happen if it was not addressed?

What is the current practice in the EBP team's setting?

What data from the EBP team's setting indicates there is a problem?

Considering all of the information above, create a concise problem statement below.

Will this be a broad or intervention EBP question?
☐ Broad   ☐ Intervention

FIGURE 3.1 Question Development Tool (Appendix B), problems section.

CALL TO ACTION

Chapter 3 provides several helpful tools for identifying and clarifying the problem. Using one or more of those approaches, drill down into the problem. Explore it from various angles and seek input from people knowledgeable about the issue.

1. Complete the first four sections of the Question Development Tool (Appendix B).
2. Then, consider the problem you have identified for your organization. Craft a problem statement that succinctly captures the important aspects of the problem.
3. Share the problem statement with others familiar with the issue for feedback.
4. Complete the fifth box on the Question Development Tool (Appendix B), writing a succinct problem statement.

DISCUSSION QUESTIONS

1. Why is it essential to accurately define the practice problem before formulating an EBP question, and what are the potential consequences of failing to do so?
2. What techniques or tools (e.g., root cause analysis, data exploration) are most effective in narrowing down and defining the practice problem? How can these methods enhance the quality of the EBP process?
3. How can interprofessional collaboration contribute to a more comprehensive understanding of the practice problem? What benefits does an interprofessional approach bring to this phase of the PET process?
4. What elements should a well-developed problem statement include to ensure it is compelling and actionable for the intended audience? How can a sense of urgency in a problem statement influence decision-making and support for EBP initiatives?
5. Reflect on a practice problem within your field or experience. What steps would you take to refine this problem into a clear, concise statement that could guide an EBP question?

A CLOSER LOOK

The Question Development Tool (Appendix B)

This form (see Figure 3.2) guides the EBP team in developing an answerable EBP question. It is meant to be fluid and dynamic as the team engages in the question development process. As the team becomes familiar with the evidence base for the topic of interest, they revisit, revise, and refine the question, search terms, search strategy, and sources of evidence.

Question Development Tool

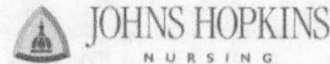

Purpose: This form guides the EBP team in developing an answerable EBP question. It is meant to be fluid and dynamic as the team engages in the question development process. As the team becomes familiar with the evidence base for the topic of interest, they revisit, revise, and refine the question, search terms, search strategy, and sources of evidence.

If viewing this online, hover over bold text for more information

What is the local problem? *(the response can be a bulleted list or phrases)*
Why is this problem important and relevant? What would happen if it was not addressed?
It is important to be able to convey the importance of addressing the issue at hand. Providing leaders and decision-makers with the drivers behind this project may help secure support.
What is the current practice in the EBP team's setting?
What data from the EBP team's setting indicates there is a problem?
In addition to highlighting why the problem is important and relevant, teams need to be able to provide data that shows the problem exists. The instructions following the tool provide some examples of sources of data such as safety, financial, quality indicators, or practice observations.
Considering all of the information above, create a concise problem statement below.
A concise statement should include the population of interest, how they are affected, and why it matters. Construct the statement as if you only had a few minutes to convey the information and get buy-in.
Will this be a broad or intervention EBP question?
☐ Broad   ☐ Intervention

FIGURE 3.2   Annotated Question Development Tool, Appendix B, p. 1.

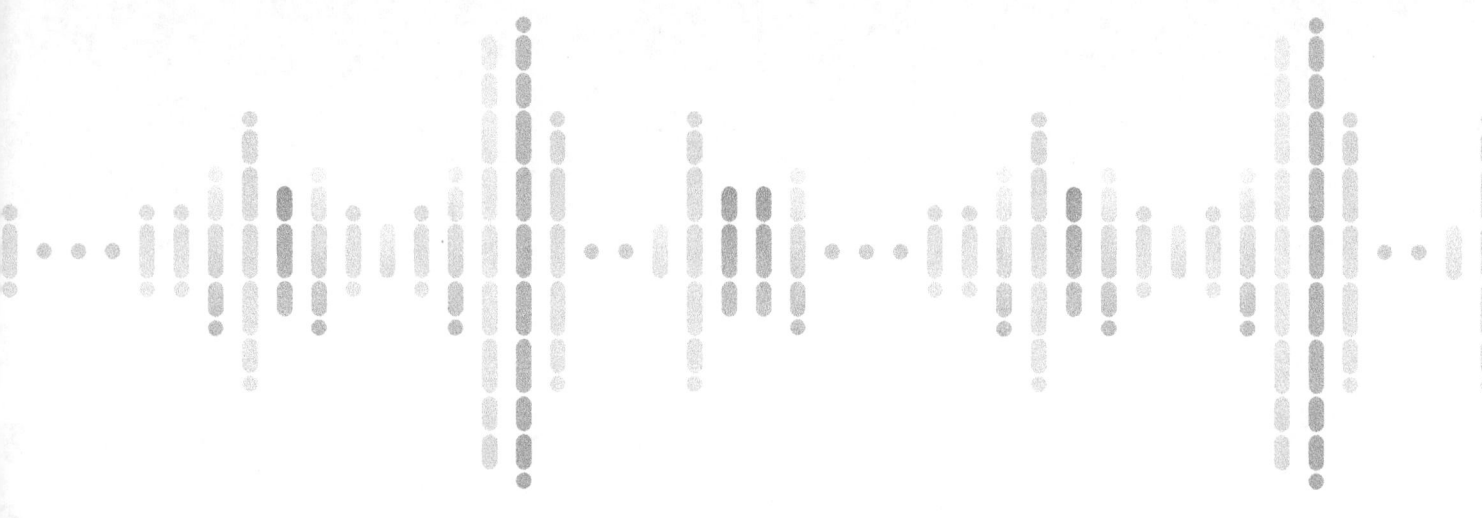

OVERVIEW

Having explored and defined the problem and developed the problem statement, the EBP team develops an answerable EBP question to address their area or topic of interest. This helps the team to understand the specific information that needs to be gathered and is used to generate a search strategy to identify evidence in the next phase—evidence. The thoughtful development of a well-structured EBP question is vital because the question drives the strategies the team will use to search for evidence. A well-defined and answerable EBP question may reduce time spent searching and increase the likelihood of finding relevant evidence. There are different types and structures of EBP questions depending on the project's starting point and objectives. This chapter provides guidance on which structures work best for a given situation.

4

PRACTICE QUESTION PHASE: THE EBP QUESTION

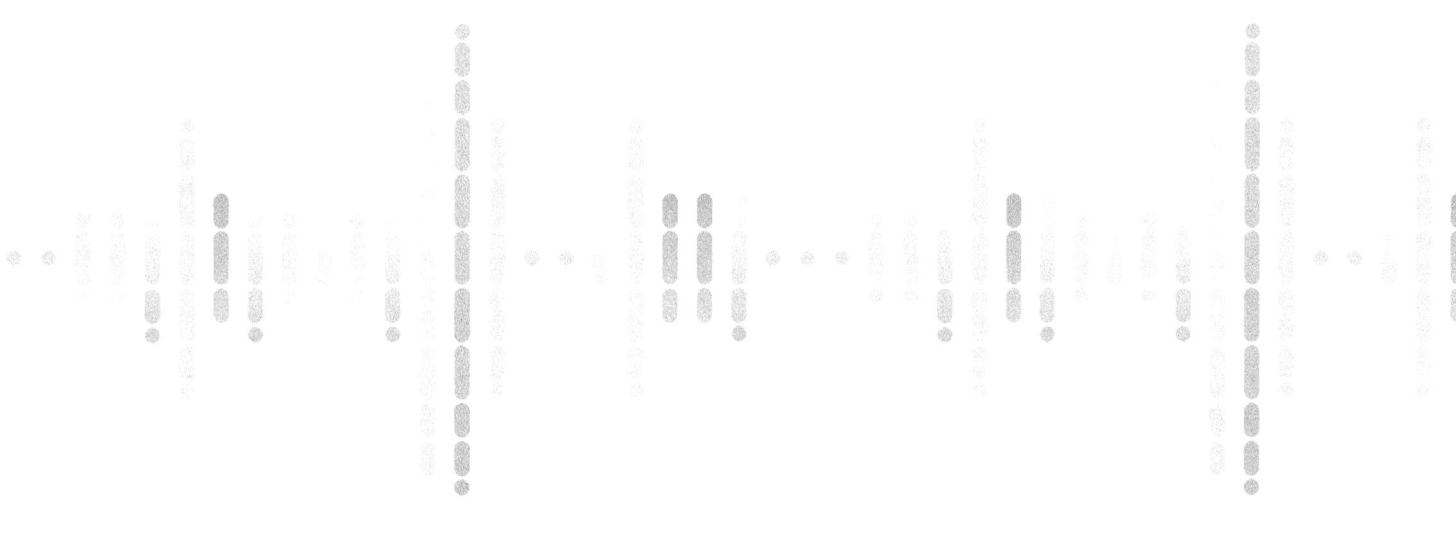

KEY POINTS

The practice question phase contains three steps. This chapter covers the final step. The JHEBP Question Development Tool (Appendix B) facilitates this step.

- In many instances, the PICO question—Patient/Population/Problem, Intervention, Comparison, and Outcome—has become synonymous with the EBP question, with teams using "PICO question" and "EBP question" interchangeably. However, PICO guides searches. It doesn't support question development as well.

- Searchable questions are concise and focused, possibly limited to two to three main ideas.

- Broad (formerly background) EBP questions cast a wide net and provide a good starting point.

- Intervention (formerly foreground) EBP questions provide more precise knowledge to drive decision-making.

- Before embarking on a full EBP project, teams should examine the project's potential alignment with organizational priorities, impact on outcomes, and ability to be implemented in the current climate.

OBJECTIVES

- 4.1 Describe a searchable question (understanding)

- 4.2 Differentiate between broad and intervention questions (analyzing)

- 4.3 Construct two types of EBP questions (creating)

LEARNING ACTIVITIES

Before completion of the learning activities, you should do the following:

- Read Chapter 4
- Listen to this podcast: https://podcasts.apple.com/us/podcast/ep-9-johns-hopkins-nursing-center-for-nursing-inquiry/id1478145611?i=1000448670860
- Review the Question Development Tool (Appendix B)

Learning Activity 4.1

What does it mean to have a searchable question? What components are important in creating a searchable question?

_____

_____

_____

_____

Learning Activity 4.2

Complete the following table, differentiating between broad and intervention questions.

	DEFINITION	PURPOSE	SEARCH YIELD	COMPONENTS
Broad				
Intervention				

Learning Activity 4.3

Part 1: Identify the relevant elements of the EBP question in the following scenario.

Central venous catheters (CVC) are necessary tools to care for critically ill children in the Pediatric Intensive Care Unit (PICU). However, improper insertion, maintenance, and removal of central lines can lead to bacterial and fungal infections, known as central line–associated bloodstream infections (CLABSIs). CLABSIs can lead to increased length of stay, healthcare costs, and morbidity and mortality.

Population:

Setting:

Topic (for broad questions) or interventions
(for intervention questions):

Outcomes (as needed):

Part 2: Now, identify the relevant elements of the EBP question in the following scenario (new information is underlined).

Central venous catheters (CVC) are necessary tools to care for critically ill children in the Pediatric Intensive Care Unit (PICU). However, improper insertion, maintenance, and removal of central lines can lead to bacterial and fungal infections, known as central line–associated bloodstream infections (CLABSIs). CLABSIs can lead to increased length of stay, healthcare costs, and morbidity and mortality. Using an equipment bundle when inserting a central line is a widespread practice to help reduce CLABSIs.

Population:

Setting:

Topic (for broad questions) or
interventions (for intervention questions):

Outcomes (as needed):

Part 3: Using the relevant elements identified above, craft a *broad* EBP question and an *intervention* EBP question.

Broad:

In/among (population and/or setting), what are the best practices/strategies/interventions for/regarding (topic)?

_____

_____

_____

Intervention:

According to the evidence, in/among (population and/or setting), what is the impact of (intervention) on (outcome)?

_____

_____

_____

Learning Activity 4.4

Read the following case study excerpts.

You work as a nurse in an adult medical/surgical unit at a small community hospital. On December 1st, Ms. J, a 68-year-old Black woman, was admitted to your unit from the emergency department for pneumonia. She had a peripheral intravenous (IV) catheter in place and was receiving IV antibiotics. She was also receiving supplemental oxygen via a nasal cannula and nebulizer treatments every four hours. Ms. J did not have any other medical conditions and was not taking any other medications.

That day, you were working the night shift, 1900 to 0700, and assigned to care for Ms. J. You received in report that Ms. J did not have a history of falls, did not require any ambulatory aids, and used her call bell for assistance. At the start of your shift, Ms. J was seated in a chair chatting with visitors. You completed your fall risk assessment using a scored screening tool, which determined that Ms. J was a low risk for falls. You also completed an environmental safety check; you did not observe any slip, trip, or fall hazards at that time. As you left the room, you instructed Ms. J to ring her call bell if she needed any assistance.

The next couple hours of your shift were busy. A new patient was admitted to your hallway from surgery. Even though you were not assigned to admit the patient, you were the most experienced nurse in your hallway and were needed as a resource.

At 2330, you heard Ms. J shouting for help from the hallway. You found Ms. J on the floor; she tripped and fell on her way to the bathroom. As you entered the room to help, you noticed multiple new environmental hazards. Since you last performed your environmental safety check, someone had added extension tubing to Ms. J's nasal cannula, and the extra tubing was tangled around her IV pole. Her visitors had also left, and there were chairs scattered about the room.

As a result of her fall, Ms. J broke her hip, which will require surgery. This will increase her hospital stay, increase her healthcare costs, and decrease her quality of life.

During your root cause analysis, you discover that Ms. J's fall is not an isolated incident. Over the past quarter, there has been a 35% increase in falls on your unit. The falls on your unit were caused by a variety of issues but most commonly occurred because of patient-related factors (e.g., age, medical conditions, medications, etc.) or environmental factors (e.g., clutter, wet floors, poor lighting, etc.).

Like all healthcare organizations, your hospital is dedicated to preventing patient falls. To prevent patient falls, your organization currently employs a scored fall risk assessment tool, an environmental safety checklist, patient education, and, when needed, wrist band identification, position alarms, and sitters.

Chart audits were performed on all charts from Q2 to determine if healthcare workers were properly documenting a patient's risk for falling, the safety of the environment, and patient education. The chart audit revealed that a fall risk assessment was properly documented 95% of the time, an environmental safety check was properly documented 92% of the time, and patient education was properly documented 86% of the time.

You begin to wonder if the interventions your hospital uses for fall prevention are still best practice and if there is anything more you can do to prevent falls in hospitalized adults.

Using the excerpts from the case study, complete the remaining sections (see Figure 4.1) of the Question Development Tool (Appendix B). For this case study, only develop a broad question.

Will this be a broad or intervention EBP question?	
☐ Broad	☐ Intervention

Identify the relevant elements of the EBP question *(some items may not be used)*	
Population	
Setting	
Topic (for broad questions) or **Intervention**(s) (for intervention questions)	
Outcomes (as needed)	

Use the information above, and the sentence templates below, to construct the EBP question.

For Broad EBP Questions:

In/among _____ , what are best practices/strategies/interventions for/regarding _____?
     (*population and/or setting*)   (*topic*)

For Intervention EBP Questions:

According to the evidence, in/among _____ , what is the impact of _____ on _____?
                               (*population and/or setting*)   (*intervention**)   (*outcome*)

*If comparing more than one intervention, provide the interventions and separate them with the phrase "as compared to"

Record the completed EBP question below.

If needed after a preliminary evidence search/review, record an updated or revised EBP question here.

FIGURE 4.1 Question Development Tool (Appendix B).

> **CALL TO ACTION**
>
> Using the problem statement your team developed, craft a searchable, broad EBP question (if appropriate, also craft an intervention question). Complete the question boxes on the Question Development Tool (Appendix B). These start with identifying if it is a broad or an intervention question.

DISCUSSION QUESTIONS

1. What are the key differences between a broad best practice question and an intervention best practice question? In what situations would an EBP team benefit from starting with a broad question rather than an intervention-focused one?

2. How does the process of framing an EBP question align with the organization's strategic goals, and why is this alignment crucial for the success of an EBP project?

3. What factors should EBP teams consider when deciding whether an EBP project is necessary or appropriate for a given practice issue? How can this decision impact the effectiveness and resource allocation of the project?

4. Why is it important to invest time in developing a well-structured, searchable question at the start of an EBP project? What are the potential long-term benefits of this approach for the E (evidence) phase?

5. Reflect on a current or past EBP project you are familiar with. How did the initial question influence the project's direction, and in hindsight, what adjustments to the question would have enhanced the project's outcomes?

A CLOSER LOOK

The Question Development Tool (Appendix B), question section

The question section (see Figure 4.2) follows the problem statement. It provides structure for the team to develop a searchable EBP question.

Will this be a broad or intervention EBP question?			
☐ Broad	Recall that broad questions should be used when the team has little knowledge of the topic or wants to understand all the available evidence.	☐ Intervention	Intervention questions are more specific and may be used to focus on one intervention or compare multiple interventions.

Identify the relevant elements of the EBP question *(some items may not be used)*

Population	
Setting	Keep in mind, broad questions typically do not have interventions or outcomes. They provide a wide spectrum of evidence on a topic.
Topic (for broad questions) or **Intervention**(s) (for intervention questions)	
Outcomes (as needed)	

Use the information above, and the sentence templates below, to construct the EBP question.

For Broad EBP Questions:

In/among _____ , what are best practices/strategies/interventions for/regarding _____ ?
     (*population and/or setting*)   (*topic*)

For Intervention EBP Questions:

According to the evidence, in/among _____ , what is the impact of _____ on _____ ?

"According to the evidence" is added to intervention questions to avoid confusion with research questions and to emphasize the search for established best practices.

and/or setting)   (*intervention**)   (*outcome*)

ide the interventions and separate them with the phrase "as compared

Record the completed EBP question below.

If needed after a preliminary evidence search/review, record an updated or revised EBP question here.

EBP teams may find the original problem statement and/or EBP question did not quite capture what the team intended. Perhaps the evidence they found was not in line with the actual problem. The team can revise the question, record it here, and move forward with the project.

FIGURE 4.2 Question section of the Question Development Tool (Appendix B).

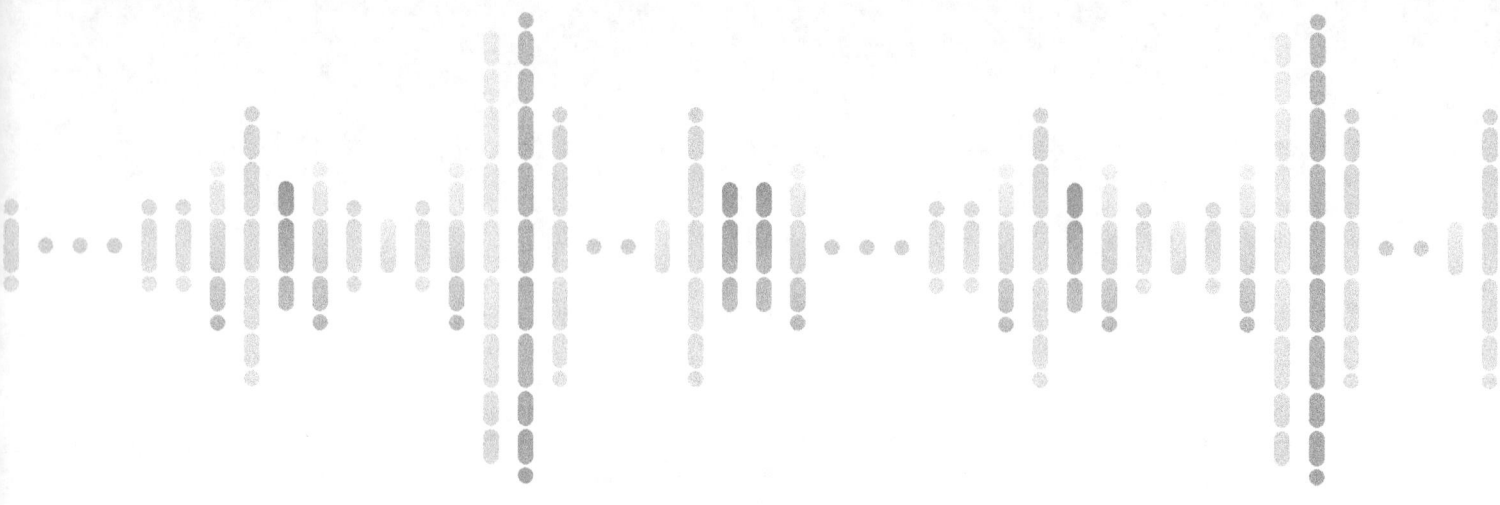

OVERVIEW

EBP requires collaboration among health professionals, who bring their diverse and specialized knowledge, skills, and methods to the project. This chapter guides the team on how to form and manage an effective interprofessional EBP team. It empowers them with the knowledge and tools to translate evidence into practice and overcome the challenges and barriers that may arise along the way.

5

THE INTERPROFESSIONAL TEAM

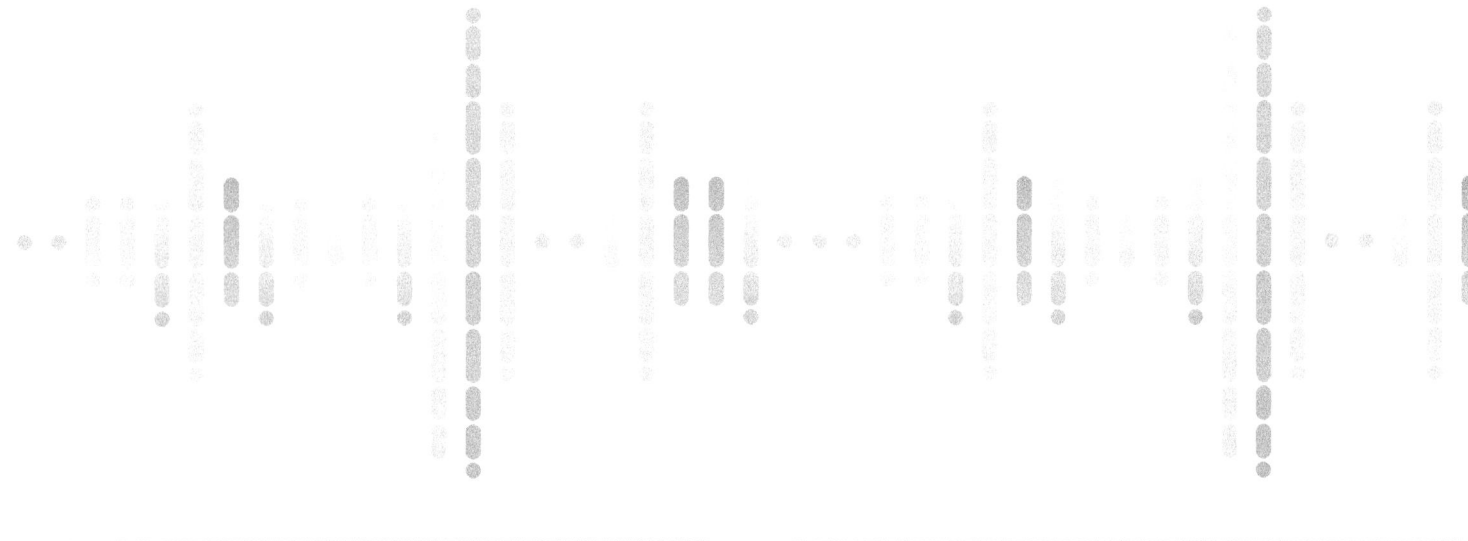

KEY POINTS

- It is critical to build an interprofessional team to collaborate with when embarking on an EBP project.

- When building core EBP team members and the team leader, consider their expertise, influence, character traits, behavior traits, and team dynamics.

- Consider impacted groups that may influence or be influenced by the EBP project. Impacted groups can include patients, families, managers, and policymakers.

- Impacted groups can broaden the team's perspective, enhance the project's impact, and make the audience feel inclusive and considerate of all perspectives.

- Recognizing and appreciating contributions within the team enhances belonging and commitment to the project.

- Successful teams tend to have a clear vision and direction.

OBJECTIVES

- 5.1 Identify impacted parties (understanding)

- 5.2 Review communication plan resource (understanding)

LEARNING ACTIVITIES

Before completion of the learning activities, you should do the following:

- Read Chapter 5
- Listen to the following podcast: https://podcasts.hopkinsmedicine.org/episode-50-engaging-staff-in-inquiry-work/
- Review the Impacted Groups Analysis and Communication Resource (Hopkins.org/resources)

Learning Activity 5.1

Identify the four roles impacted groups may fill and define.

1. _____

2. _____

3. _____

4. _____

Learning Activity 5.2

Read the following case study excerpt.

After defining your problem and formulating your EBP question, it's time to examine your impacted parties. You start by brainstorming a list of anyone who may influence or be influenced by the EBP project. Here's a snapshot of your list:

Sofia is a clinical nurse specialist on your unit. She is well respected by staff and valued for her clinical experience and expertise. She has led multiple quality improvement initiatives on the unit and is a staunch advocate for patient safety.

Ravi is a third-party vendor. He is contracted by your hospital to provide medical equipment and supplies.

Liam is the environmental services team lead. He supervises and leads the team of environmental services technicians that maintain your unit.

Sam is a hospital pharmacist. He was instrumental in launching the STEADI-Rx initiative at your hospital, which provides guidance to pharmacists on how to screen pharmacy patients, assess their medications, and intervene to reduce fall risk.

Mei is a bedside nurse. She has been a nurse on your unit for 23 years and is very involved in unit-based activities. She is on the Comprehensive Unit Based Safety Committee, is a fall safety champion, and frequently precepts newer nurses. She was in charge the night Ms. J fell.

Lee is your nurse manager. They foster an environment that is supportive of inquiry and fully endorse your EBP project. However, due to time constraints, they are unable to help out with the day-to-day tasks of the project.

Using the excerpt from the case study, complete the Impacted Groups Analysis portion (see Figure 5.1) of the Impacted Groups Analysis and Communication Resource. Recall that roles may be filled by more than one individual or group.

Impacted Groups Analysis	
Identify the key impacted groups:	
☐ Manager or direct supervisor ☐ Finance department ☐ Vendors ☐ Patients and/or families; patient and family advisory committee ☐ Professional organizations ☐ Committees	☐ Organizational leaders ☐ Interdisciplinary colleagues (e.g., physicians, nutritionists, respiratory therapists, or OT/PT) ☐ Administrators ☐ Other units or departments ☐ Others: _____

Impacted Groups Analysis Matrix: (Adapted from http://www.tools4dev.org/)

Impacted Individual/Group Name and Title:	Role: (select all that apply) Responsibility, Approval, Consult, Inform	Impact Level: How much does the project impact them? (minor, moderate, significant)	Influence Level: How much influence do they have over the project? (minor, moderate, significant)	What matters most to the indivual or group?	How could they contribute to the project?	How could they impede the project?	Strategy(s) for engaging them:

FIGURE 5.1 Impacted Groups Analysis and Communication Resource.

> **CALL TO ACTION**
>
> If you have not done so yet, build your EBP team and identify a team leader. Consider the impacted parties. Make a list of groups or individuals relevant to your project. Identify potential strengths and barriers. Use the Impacted Groups Analysis and Communication Resource (Hopkins.org/resources) to help outline your approach.

DISCUSSION QUESTIONS

1. What are the essential qualities or skills that EBP team leaders should possess to effectively lead an interprofessional team? How can these qualities contribute to the team's overall success?

2. In what ways can diverse healthcare professionals contribute unique perspectives to an EBP project? What are some strategies to ensure that all voices and specialties are heard and valued within the team?

3. How can EBP teams identify and involve relevant impacted groups outside of the core team? What benefits do these groups bring to the EBP process, and how can their involvement enhance project outcomes?

4. What are some common challenges interprofessional EBP teams may face, and what strategies can be employed to overcome these obstacles to maintain effective teamwork and engagement?

5. How can interprofessional EBP teams establish and maintain accountability throughout the project? What tools or methods might help sustain team motivation and commitment to the project's goals?

A CLOSER LOOK

Impacted Groups Analysis and Communication Resource

This resource (see Figure 5.2) prompts teams to identify potential impacted groups and plan communication. It is not meant to be completed only at one time point but referenced throughout the project.

Impacted Groups Analysis

Identify the key impacted groups:

- ☐ Manager or direct supervisor
- ☐ Finance department
- ☐ Vendors
- ☐ Patients and/or families; patient and family advisory committee
- ☐ Professional organizations
- ☐ Committees
- ☐ Organizational leaders
- ☐ Interdisciplinary colleagues (e.g., physicians, nutritionists, respiratory therapists, or OT/PT)
- ☐ Administrators
- ☐ Other units or departments
- ☐ Others: _____

Impacted Groups Analysis Matrix: (Adapted from http://www.tools4dev.org/)

Impacted Individual/Group Name and Title:	Role: (select all that apply) Responsibility, Approval, Consult, Inform	Impact Level: How much does the project impact them? (minor, moderate, significant)	Influence Level: How much influence do they have over the project? (minor, moderate, significant)	What matters most to the indivual or group?	How could they contribute to the project?	How could they impede the project?	Strategy(s) for engaging them:

> *One individual or group may have more than one role.*

> *The team should identify people with a vested interest, role, and/or responsibility in the project. For example, approval of a policy may fall to unit leaders, whereas clinicians may provide consultation on feasibility.*

> *Spending time identifying the potential contributions and impediments of each individual or group helps the team strategize for a successful implementation.*

Communication Planning

Refer to this section to guide your communications t[o...]

> *The reporting section may be helpful at any stage of the process but is particularly useful when the team is ready to disseminate their findings. The three most important messages may only be evident once recommendations are determined. However, teams can use this structure to develop and tailor any type of communication.*

What is the purpose of the dissemination of the EBP p[roject?]
- ☐ Raise awareness
- ☐ Promote action
- ☐ Change policy
- ☐ Change p[ractice]
- ☐ Engage i[n...]

What are the 3 most important messages?

Align key message(s) and methods with the audience:

> *Teams should consider multiple modalities for communicating the key messages. Think of delivering them multiple times and in multiple ways.*

Audience	Key Messages		Timing
Interdisciplinary groups			
Organizational leadership			
Frontline nurses			
Departmental leadership			
External community			
Other			

> *Align the key message with the audience. People are interested in what change means to them and how they may be affected. Refer back to the matrix to see what each impacted individual values. Carefully tailoring the message to the audience ensures their concerns are met.*

FIGURE 5.2 Impacted Groups Analysis and Communication Resource, annotated.

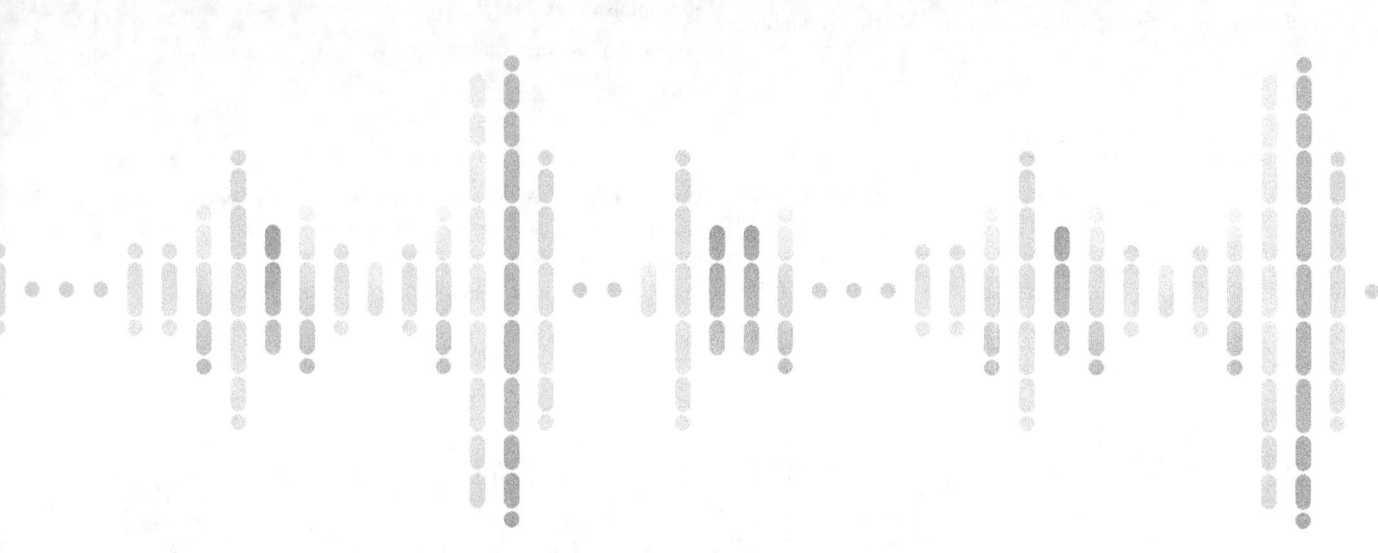

OVERVIEW

Finding and evaluating evidence, the cornerstone of evidence-based healthcare, is the second phase of the JHEBP PET process. The team uses the EBP question generated in the previous phase to guide their collection and selection of evidence. This chapter describes what types of evidence the team may find during their exploration of the literature. This will lay the foundation for the next steps in the EBP process, which include searching for evidence, screening the results, and appraising the applicable literature. Understanding these various types of evidence is crucial, as each contributes uniquely to the overall picture of best practices. For instance, qualitative studies offer insights into patient experiences and perspectives, while quantitative studies provide measurable data on treatment outcomes. Systematic reviews synthesize existing studies to present comprehensive conclusions, and clinical guidelines offer evidence-based recommendations for practice.

6

EVIDENCE PHASE: INTRODUCTION TO EVIDENCE

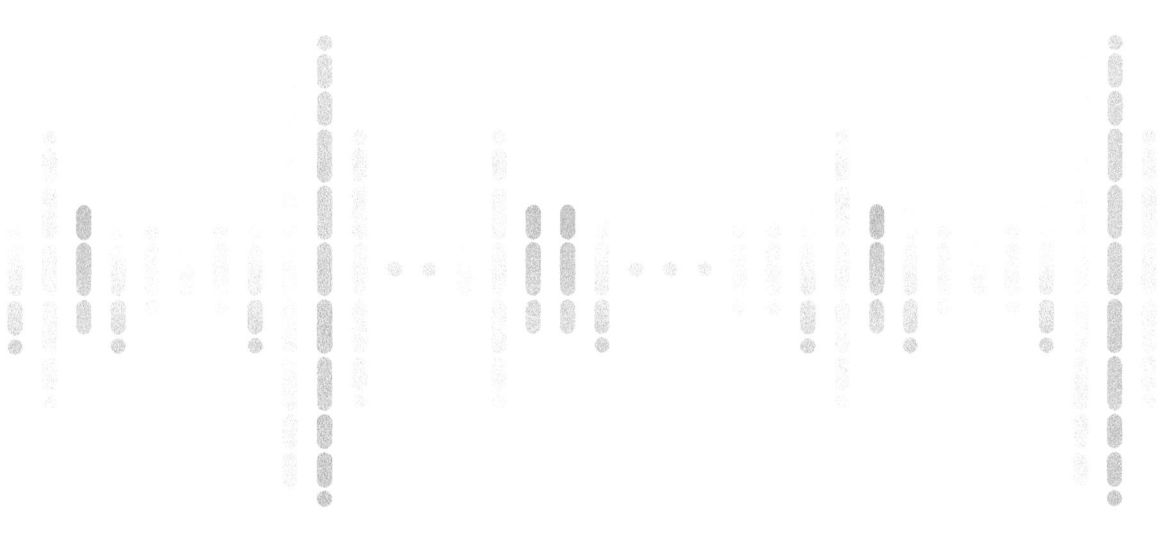

KEY POINTS

The evidence phase contains seven steps. This chapter gives an overview of the evidence gathered and appraised in Steps 4, 5, and 6. Information in this chapter will assist the EBP team in completing the JHEBP Pre-appraised Evidence Appraisal Tool, Single Study Evidence Appraisal Tool, and Anecdotal Evidence Appraisal Tool (Appendices E1, E2, and E3, respectively).

- The JHEBP model has updated its approach to evidence appraisal.

- Pre-appraised evidence—such as clinical practice guidelines, literature reviews with a systematic approach, and evidence summaries—can provide independent support for decision-making if they are suitable to the EBP problem and of sufficient quality.

- There are various types of literature reviews with a systematic approach, but all must meet specific criteria to be considered "systematic."

- Single studies with formal study designs can provide strong or moderate support for decision-making if they are of sufficient quality.

- Studies may follow qualitative, quantitative, or mixed-methods approaches.

- Anecdotal evidence—such as expert opinions, book chapters, position statements, case reports, programmatic experiences, and literature reviews without a systematic approach—provides limited support for decision-making.

OBJECTIVES

- 6.1 Differentiate between the main types of evidence (analyzing)

- 6.2 Describe support for decision-making (understanding)

- 6.3 Select appropriate approaches to generate evidence (evaluating)

LEARNING ACTIVITIES

Before completion of the learning activities, you should do the following:

- Read Chapter 6
- Listen to this podcast: https://podcasts.apple.com/us/podcast/ep20-johns-hopkins-center-for-nursing-inquiry-different/id1478145611?i=1000480879172
- Download the Evidence Terminology and Considerations Guide (Appendix F; Hopkins.org/tools)

Learning Activity 6.1

Align the descriptions with the appropriate type of evidence. Write the letters of the corresponding descriptions in the appropriate boxes.

PRE-APPRAISED EVIDENCE	a. uses systematic inquiry to answer questions or solve problems
	b. allows clinicians to rely on the expertise of content and research methods experts to process literature and generate recommendations
	c. categorized by the design, not the intent
	d. serves as independent support for decision-making in healthcare
SINGLE STUDIES	e. published information that was not generated from a research study but rather from personal, professional, or clinical experience
	f. examples include clinical practice guidelines, literature reviews with a systematic approach, and evidence summaries
	g. types include expert opinion, case report, programmatic experience, and literature review without a systematic approach
	h. studies that have undergone a methodical process for collection and critical evaluation
ANECDOTAL EVIDENCE	i. can be categorized by both the methodologic approach (quantitative, qualitative, or mixed-methods) and the design
	j. provides low support for decision-making
	k. scientific data in the form of qualitative and quantitative data
	l. also known as filtered or secondary literature

Learning Activity 6.2

Part 1: Describe support for decision-making.

_____

_____

_____

Part 2: Identify the degree of support for decision-making provided by these types of evidence.

Pre-appraised evidence

Single studies with formal study designs

Anecdotal evidence

Learning Activity 6.3

Circle the appropriate approaches to generate evidence for each scenario below.

1. Researchers are trying to gain an in-depth understanding of online gaming addiction in adolescents, including opinions, meanings, and motivations. Little has been explored on this topic, so they hope to generate some hypotheses and directions for further study. The researchers would be best served to conduct:

    a. A quantitative study to understand the scope of the problem in actual numbers

    b. A qualitative study to thoroughly explore the issue and bring meaning to a fairly new phenomenon

    c. A mixed-methods study to explore the phenomenon from all aspects and focus on more specific pieces of the problem

2. A research team has developed a new device to prevent pressure injuries in hospitalized adults. They need to determine how effective this device is in preventing injury. They need to conduct:

    a. A qualitative study to understand how patients feel about the device and learn about their experiences with pressure injuries

    b. A mixed-methods study to both measure the effectiveness of the device and understand nurses' thoughts on pressure injury prevention

    c. A quantitative study to generate numerical data reflecting the effectiveness of the device

3. Researchers would like to determine if a structured RN-to-RN handoff works to convey important patient care issues and identify any barriers that may exist to prevent its full-scale adoption. They should conduct:

    a. A mixed-methods study using a quantitative measure of the number of patient care issues conveyed and interviews with staff to understand any barriers to providing this type of handoff

    b. A qualitative study to define handoff and explore potential barriers experienced by nurses

    c. A quantitative study looking at the number of patient care issues conveyed through the handoff process

CALL TO ACTION

Let's pause here a moment to refer back to the EBP Project Steps and Overview (Appendix A), specifically the evidence decision tree (back side; see Figure 6.1). Begin by determining if your EBP question fits with organizational priorities. If it does, continue moving forward. If it does not, take some time to determine alternatives, identify other solutions, or reexamine the problem.

DISCUSSION QUESTIONS

1. How does the Johns Hopkins EBP model define "evidence" within the context of EBP, and why is it important for EBP teams to clearly understand this definition?

2. What are the key types of evidence that an EBP team might encounter, and how can each type contribute uniquely to addressing a practice question?

3. What recent changes to the Johns Hopkins EBP model influence how evidence is assessed, and how do these changes reflect advancements in evidence-based healthcare?

4. Why is it crucial for EBP teams to align their assessment methods with contemporary standards and practices in healthcare, and what impact might this alignment have on patient care outcomes?

5. During the literature search, what methods can EBP teams employ to efficiently screen and appraise different types of evidence? How do these methods ensure the selection of high-quality, relevant evidence?

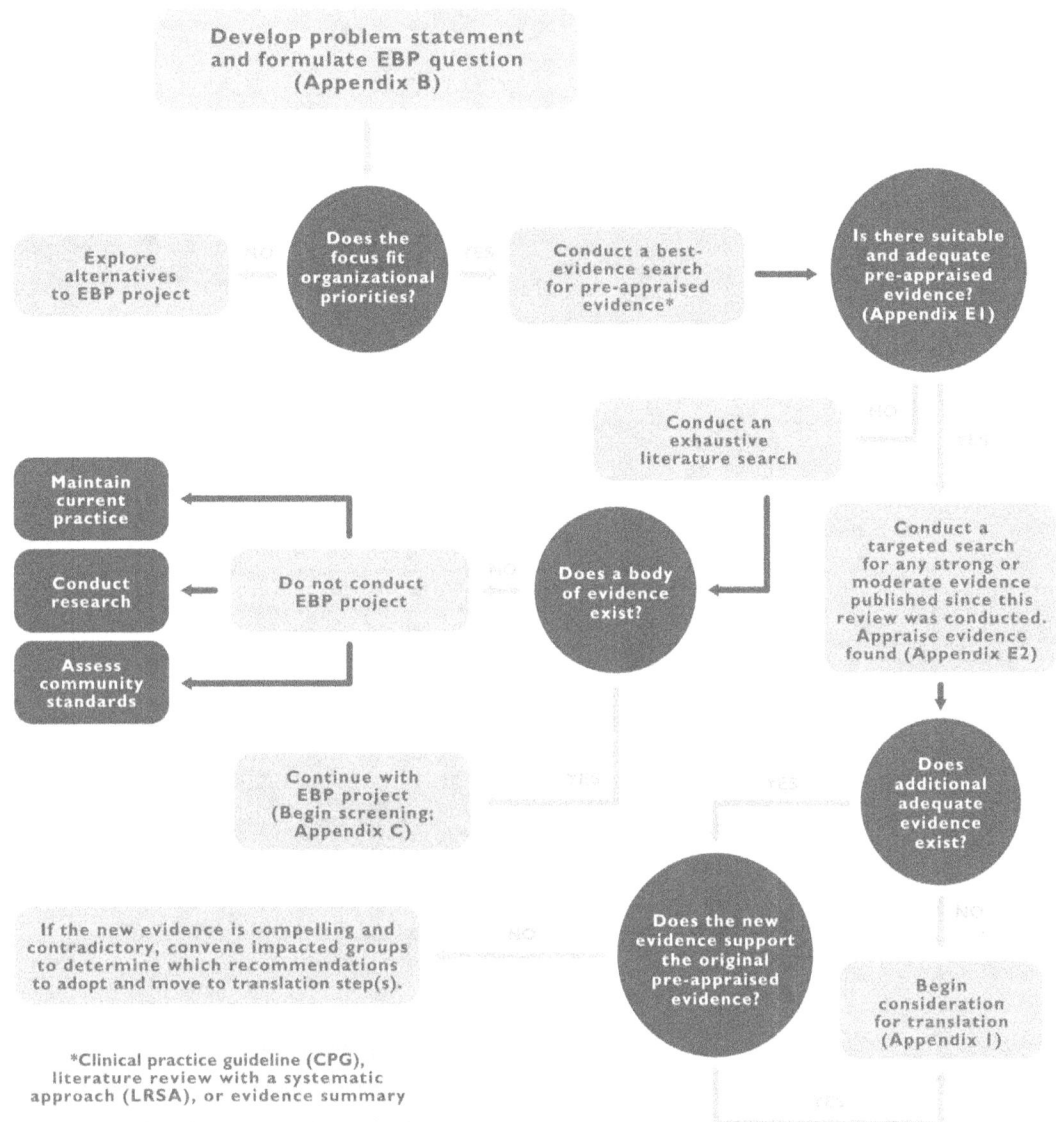

FIGURE 6.1 Evidence decision tree (Appendix A).

A CLOSER LOOK

The Evidence Terminology and Considerations Guide (Appendix F)

This tool (see Figure 6.2) serves as a glossary of important terms found in the appraisal tools. All bolded terms from the appraisal tools (Appendices E1, E2, and E3) are included in the table along with definitions and context.

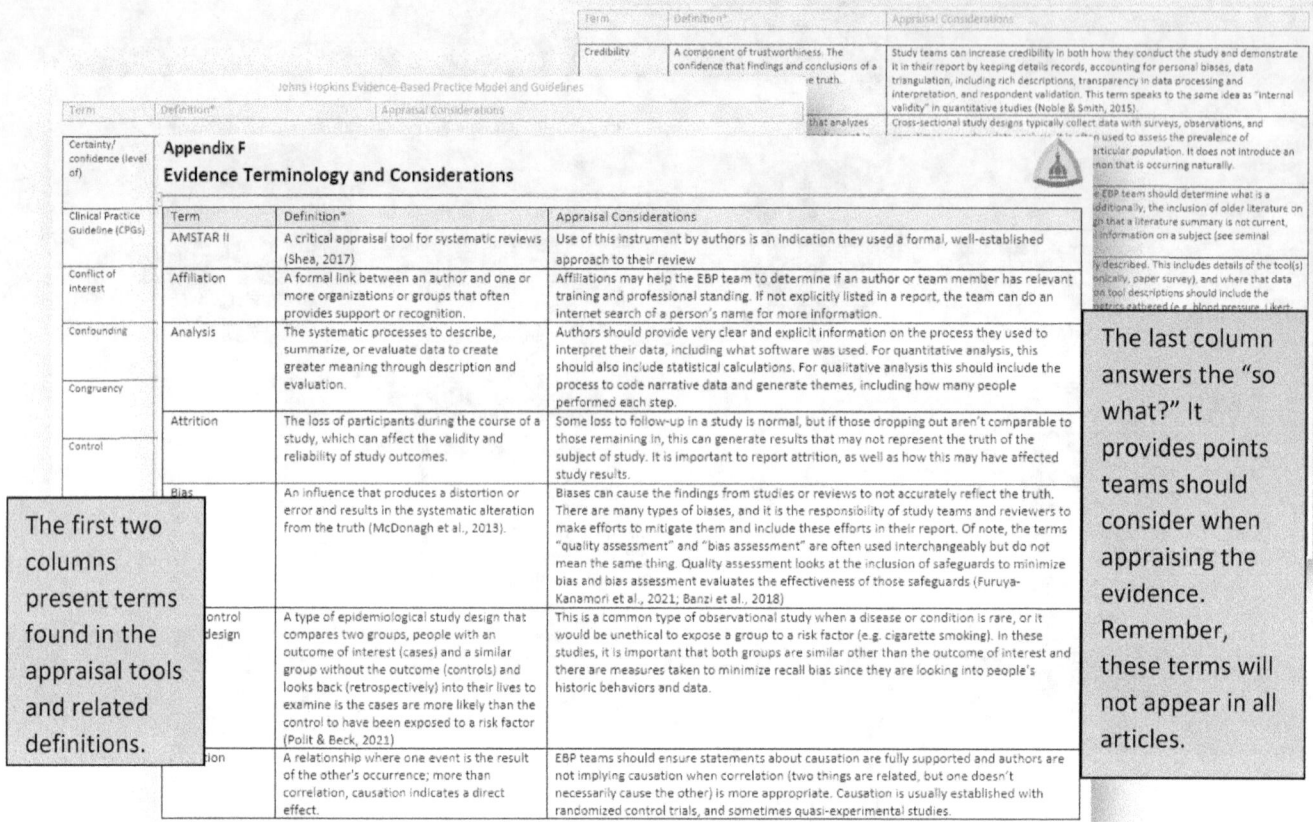

FIGURE 6.2 Evidence Terminology and Considerations Guide (Appendix F), annotated.

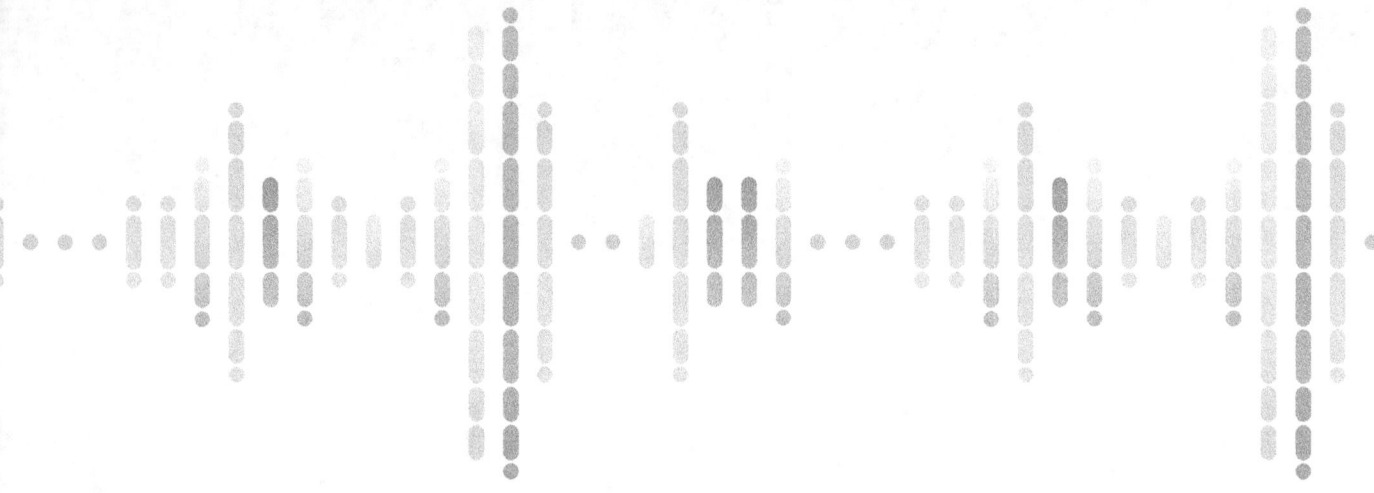

OVERVIEW

This chapter reviews types of literature searches; when, where, and how to conduct them; and the process of screening results to generate an accurate and manageable representation of the literature. The goal of these steps is to identify actionable information in the most efficient way possible. This may be in the form of accessible pre-appraised evidence or through an EBP team's own exhaustive literature search to find answers to their EBP question. Finally, as with all healthcare decisions, the team should be cautious of introducing biases while collecting evidence and the potential this has to perpetuate skewed perspectives.

7

EVIDENCE PHASE: THE EVIDENCE SEARCH AND SCREENING

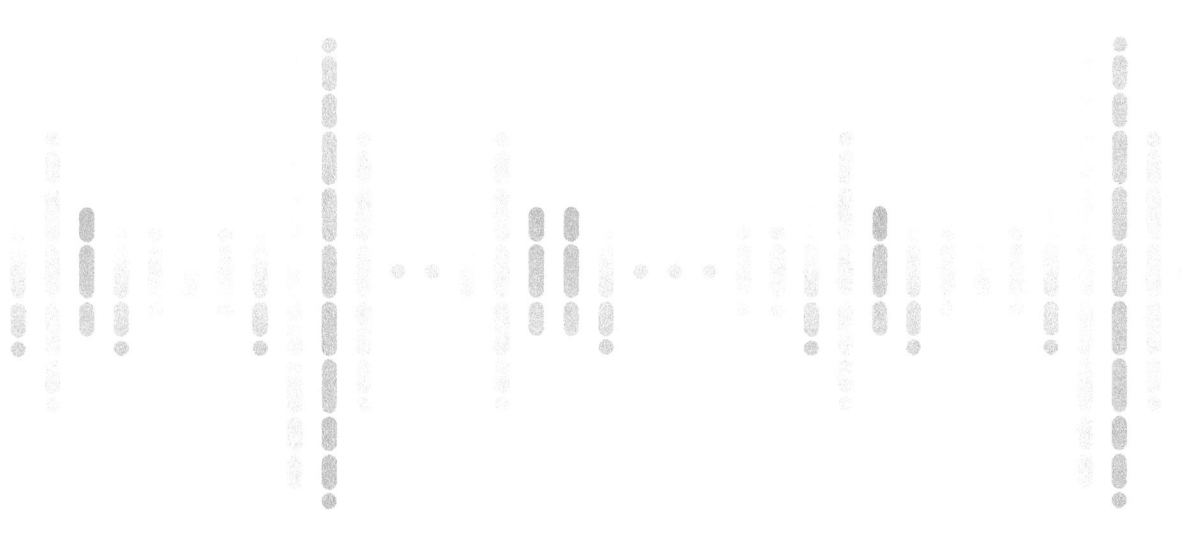

KEY POINTS

The evidence phase contains seven steps. This chapter covers the first two. The JHEBP Searching and Screening Tool (Appendix C) facilitates these steps.

- There are various types of literature searches an EBP team can conduct, yet all should follow a systematic process to promote efficiency and minimize bias.

- Best-evidence literature searches concentrate on gathering foundational information and pre-appraised evidence. Various databases specialize in providing this type of evidence.

- Exhaustive evidence literature searches attempt to gather all literature on a topic within pre-determined parameters. EBP teams design search strategies to conduct these searches.

- The EBP question guides the literature search. EBP teams will need to isolate the elements of their EBP question to create search concepts and build search strings.

- Additional tools to create search strings include truncation, Boolean operators, controlled vocabulary, exact phrasing, and title/abstract limiters.

- Literature screening is a systematic process to winnow down the results of an exhaustive search in an unbiased manner to only those that answer the EBP question and meet inclusion/exclusion criteria.

- Documenting the search and screening process is an important element to establish rigor and replicability.

- Various forms of bias can influence the trustworthiness of the results of a team's literature search. Bias should be recognized and minimized.

OBJECTIVES

- 7.1 Differentiate between a best-evidence search and an exhaustive search (analyzing)

- 7.2 Develop a replicable search string (applying)

- 7.3 Identify ways to screen evidence (understanding)

LEARNING ACTIVITIES

Before completion of the learning activities, you should do the following:

- Read Chapter 7
- Listen to this podcast: https://podcasts.apple.com/us/podcast/episode-55-searching-pre-appraised-evidence-part-1/id1478145611?i=1000658675607
- Listen to this podcast: https://podcasts.apple.com/us/podcast/episode-56-who-produces-sources-of-pre-appraised/id1478145611?i=1000658675608
- Listen to this podcast: https://podcasts.apple.com/us/podcast/episode-57-repositories-of-pre-appraised-evidence/id1478145611?i=1000658675782
- Download the Searching and Screening Tool (Appendix C; Hopkins.org/tools)

Learning Activity 7.1

Part 1: Differentiate between a best-evidence search and an exhaustive search.

TYPE OF SEARCH	DEFINITION	BEST USE
Best-evidence		
Exhaustive		

Part 2: Name three sources of best evidence.

1. _____

2. _____

3. _____

Learning Activity 7.2

Part 1: Fill out the elements in Figure 7.1—section I of the Searching and Screening Tool (Appendix C).

Section I: Key Elements of the EBP Question	
Identify the key elements of the EBP question (*from the Question Development Tool*)	
Population	
Setting	
Topic or Intervention(s)	
Outcomes (as needed)	

FIGURE 7.1 Searching and Screening Tool (Appendix C), section I.

Part 2: Conduct a best-evidence search (see Figure 7.2) using those key elements identified in part 1. Search some of the sources for pre-appraised evidence such as the Cochrane Library, JBI, National Institutes of Health and Care Excellence (NICE), US Preventative Services Taskforce (USPSTF), Agency for Healthcare Research and Quality (AHRQ), World Health Organization (WHO), and professional organizations. Were you able to find a clinical practice guideline, literature review with a systematic approach, or evidence summary? If so, you could appraise the evidence and move to a targeted search. However, for this exercise we will move to an exhaustive search.

Section II: Best-Evidence Search
Does pre-appraised evidence exist in the form of clinical practice guidelines (CPGs), literature reviews with a systematic approach (LRSAs), or evidence summaries?
☐ Yes → Appraise using the Pre-appraised Evidence Appraisal Tool (Appendix E1) 　　○ Is the evidence suitable and of adequate quality? 　　　☐ Yes → Complete targeted search for additional evidence based on search date in pre-appraised evidence to determine if relevant evidence has been published in the interim 　　　☐ No → Skip to Section III (Exhaustive Search) ☐ No → Skip to Section III (Exhaustive Search)

FIGURE 7.2 Searching and Screening Tool (Appendix C), section II.

Part 3: Complete the provided sections of the Searching and Screening Tool (Appendix C; see Figure 7.3).

Section III: Exhaustive Search and Screening	
Complete the table below using the population, setting, topic or intervention(s), and outcomes identified in Section I. List the element and associated terms to build a full search concept.	
EBP Question Element	Possible Search Terms (*synonyms, alternative spellings, or brand names*)
1)	
2)	
3)	
What databases will you search? ☐ CINAHL ☐ PsychINFO ☐ MEDLINE (PubMed) ☐ Epistemonikos ☐ Embase ☐ Other:	
What are the inclusion and exclusion criteria?	
Inclusion:	Exclusion:
What date limit will you use and why?	

FIGURE 7.3 Searching and Screening Tool (Appendix C), section III.

Part 4: Using the information you gathered above, spend some time developing a replicable search string for at least one database. Conduct the search and record the number of articles you found (see Figure 7.4).

What are the search strings and number of results from each database?		
Database	Search String	Number of Results

FIGURE 7.4 Searching and Screening Tool (Appendix C), section III, part 3.

Learning Activity 7.3

Identify two ways the team can effectively screen the evidence from the searches.

1. _____

_____

2. _____

_____

Learning Activity 7.4

Complete the screening flow chart based on the provided scenario.

The EBP team searched three databases—CINAHL, PubMed, and Embase—and found 230 articles to review. Team members additionally uncovered six articles through hand searching. The team reviewed the collected evidence and found and removed 23 duplicate articles. From a title and abstract screening of the remaining articles, five were removed because they were not in English, seven discussed children and not adults, 43 were not on topic, and 26 were excluded because they fell well outside the year limits. Subsequent full-text screening excluded 25 articles that used an alternative intervention that was not the focus of this project, 25 that were based on children, and four that were not retrievable as full text.

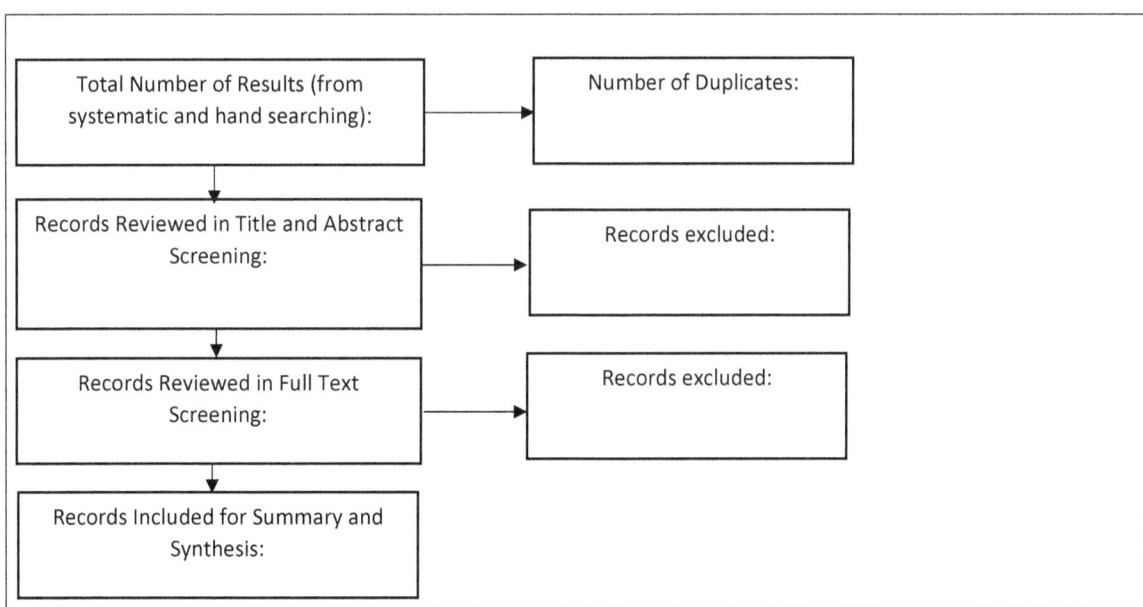

CALL TO ACTION

Let's focus on the Searching and Screening Tool (Appendix C).

Assuming your EBP focus fits organizational priorities, you are now ready to begin searching. First, complete section I of the Searching and Screening Tool using the EBP question developed for your project.

Then, using these key elements, conduct a best-evidence search. Recall that this type of search looks specifically for pre-appraised evidence (clinical practice guidelines, literature reviews with a systematic approach, and evidence summaries). Based on your results, complete section II (see Figure 7.5).

Section II: Best-Evidence Search
Does pre-appraised evidence exist in the form of clinical practice guidelines (CPGs), literature reviews with a systematic approach (LRSAs), or evidence summaries?
☐ Yes → Appraise using the Pre-appraised Evidence Appraisal Tool (Appendix E1) 　　o Is the evidence suitable and of adequate quality? 　　　　☐ Yes → Complete targeted search for additional evidence based on search date in pre-appraised evidence to determine if relevant evidence has been published in the interim 　　　　☐ No → Skip to Section III (Exhaustive Search) ☐ No → Skip to Section III (Exhaustive Search)

FIGURE 7.5 Searching and Screening Tool (Appendix C), section II.

If you found pre-appraised evidence, you will want to move to appraising that evidence (see the "Call to Action" section in Chapter 8 of this workbook). If the pre-appraised evidence is suitable and of high-quality, conduct a targeted search for any relevant evidence published in the interim. If new evidence aligns with the findings of the pre-appraised evidence, you can move toward translation. If the new evidence is contradictory, convene your team to determine the next steps.

If you were unable to find suitable pre-appraised evidence, conduct an exhaustive search. Identify associated terms based on your key elements. Establish inclusion and exclusion criteria and decide where to search. Complete section III (see Figure 7.6).

Section III: Exhaustive Search and Screening	
Complete the table below using the population, setting, topic or intervention(s), and outcomes identified in Section I. List the element and associated terms to build a full search concept.	
EBP Question Element	Possible Search Terms (*synonyms, alternative spellings, or brand names*)
1)	
2)	
3)	

What databases will you search?
☐ CINAHL   ☐ PsychINFO ☐ MEDLINE (PubMed)   ☐ Epistemonikos ☐ Embase   ☐ Other:
What are the inclusion and exclusion criteria?
Inclusion: Exclusion:
What date limit will you use and why?
What is the date the team conducted the search?

What are the search strings and number of results from each database?		
Database	Search String	Number of Results

How will the team systematically screen the results to identify evidence that answers the EBP question and meets the inclusion/exclusion criteria (*select all that apply*)?
☐ Use software or web-based program to track (e.g., Google Forms, Excel, Abstrackr) ☐ Have at least two independent reviewers for each record ☐ Inclusion or exclusion disagreements resolved by third reviewer ☐ Other:
Complete the screening flow chart below

FIGURE 7.6 Searching and Screening Tool (Appendix C), section III.

Once you have finished searching, screen the results using one of the methods described in the chapter. Enter your results into the flow chart (from Learning Activity 7.4).

DISCUSSION QUESTIONS

1. What are the different types of literature searches, and how can an EBP team determine which type is most suitable for addressing their specific EBP question?

2. What strategies can EBP teams use to efficiently process and screen search results to ensure they are left with a manageable and accurate representation of the literature?

3. How does the selection between pre-appraised evidence and a comprehensive literature search affect the outcomes of an EBP project? What are the advantages and limitations of each approach?

4. In what ways might biases be introduced during the literature search and screening process, and what steps can the EBP team take to minimize these biases?

5. Why is it essential for EBP teams to be vigilant about potential biases in the evidence collection phase, and what impact could these biases have on the final recommendations and patient care outcomes?

A CLOSER LOOK

The Searching and Screening Tool (Appendix C)

This tool (see Figure 7.7) guides the team through the steps of searching for evidence that answers their EBP question and tracking the process. The team will first look for pre-appraised evidence in a best-evidence search. The results of that investigation will guide the next steps (a targeted or exhaustive search). Recording the evidence identification process creates confidence in the eventual project recommendations by demonstrating a thorough and unbiased approach.

Section I: Key Elements of the EBP Question	
Identify the key elements of the EBP question (*from the Question Development Tool*)	
Population	
Setting	
Topic or Intervention(s)	
Outcomes (as needed)	

> Copy forward the key elements identified on the Question Development Tool. Recall that broad questions include population, setting, and topic. They often lack the intervention and outcome found in intervention questions.

Section II: Best-Evidence Search
Does pre-appraised evidence exist in the form of clinical practice guidelines (CPGs), literature reviews with a systematic approach (LRSAs), or evidence summaries?

☐ Yes → Appraise using the Pre-appraised Evidence Appraisal Tool (Appendix E1)
    o Is the evidence suitable and of adequate quality?
        ☐ Yes → Complete targeted search for additional evidence based on search date in pre-appraised evidence to determine if relevant evidence has been published in the interim
        ☐ No → Skip to Section III (Exhaustive Search)
 	
☐ No → Skip to Section III (Exhaustive Search)

> If a piece of pre-appraised evidence exists, it is important to determine suitability and quality before moving on.

7 EVIDENCE PHASE: THE EVIDENCE SEARCH AND SCREENING

Section III: Exhaustive Search and Screening

Complete the table below using the population, setting, topic or intervention(s), and outcomes identified in Section I. List the element and associated terms to build a full search concept.

EBP Question Element	Possible Search Terms (*synonyms, alternative spellings, or brand names*)
1)	
2)	
3)	

The team develops search terms for each key element identified. They should consider alternate names or spellings, synonyms, or brand names.

What databases will you search?

- [ ] CINAHL
- [ ] MEDLINE (PubMed)
- [ ] Embase
- [ ] PsychINFO
- [ ] Epistemonikos
- [ ] Other:

What are the inclusion and exclusion criteria?

Inclusion:	Exclusion:

Some considerations may be type of evidence, year of publication, language, population, or more specifics of the intervention.

What date limit will you use and why?

What is the date the team conducted the search?

Remember, date parameters are topic-specific and require justification. Teams should not choose an arbitrary five-year limit without rationale.

What are the search strings and number of results from each database?

Database	Search String	Number of Results

Copy and paste the search string here.

How will the team systematically screen the results to identify evidence that answers the EBP question and meets the inclusion/exclusion criteria (*select all that apply*)?

- [ ] Use software or web-based program to track (e.g., Google Forms, Excel, Abstrackr)
- [ ] Have at least two independent reviewers for each record
- [ ] Inclusion or exclusion disagreements resolved by third reviewer
- [ ] Other:

This should be a systematic and unbiased approach.

Complete the screening flow chart below

continues

(cont'd)

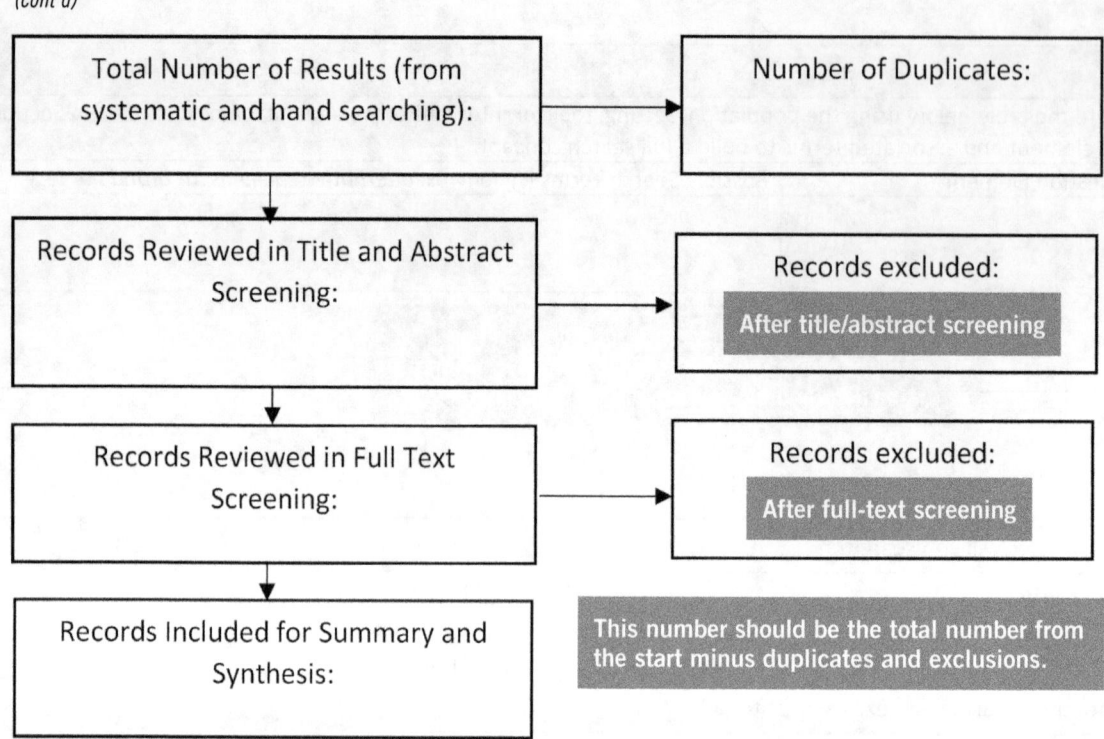

FIGURE 7.7 Searching and Screening Tool (Appendix C), annotated.

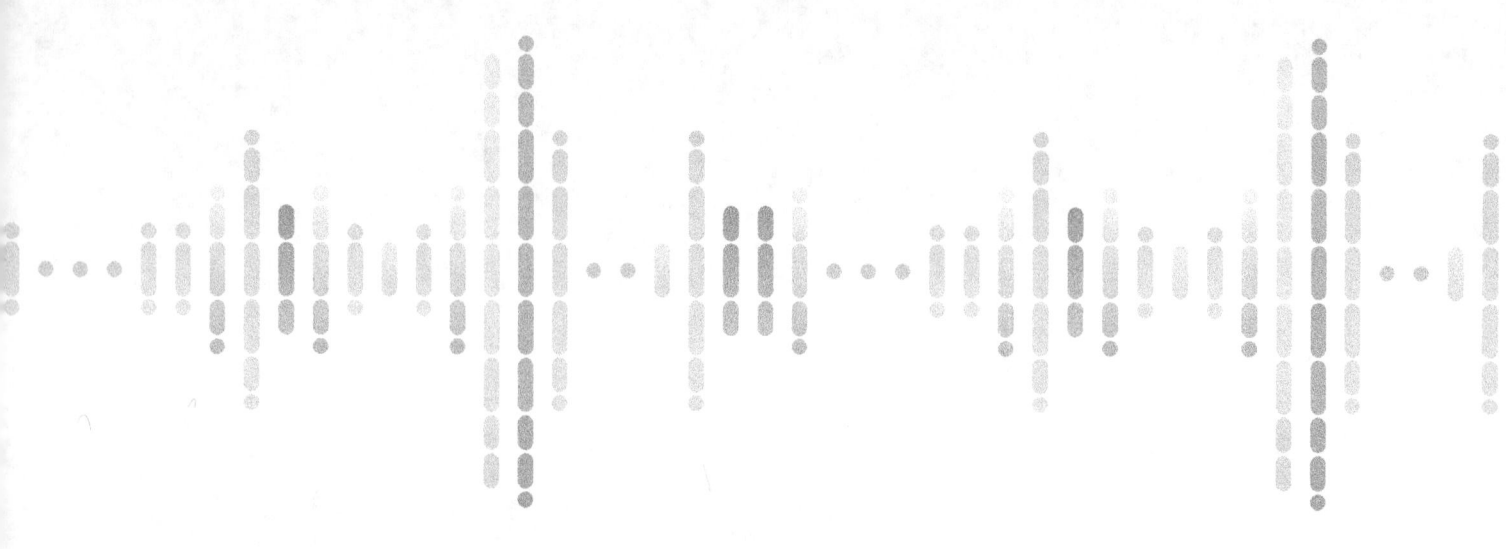

OVERVIEW

This chapter describes determining if and how evidence can inform an EBP team's decision-making. It outlines the overall purpose and methodology of the appraisal process, emphasizing special considerations for each type of evidence. These steps ensure that the team advances with sound evidence, preparing them for the subsequent steps of summarizing, synthesizing, and generating best-evidence recommendations.

8

EVIDENCE PHASE: APPRAISING THE EVIDENCE

KEY POINTS

The evidence phase contains seven steps. This chapter discusses Step 6. The JHEBP Appraisal Tool Selection Algorithm (Appendix D), Pre-appraised Evidence Appraisal Tool (Appendix E1), Single Study Evidence Appraisal Tool (Appendix E2), Anecdotal Evidence Appraisal Tool (Appendix E3), and Evidence Terminology and Considerations Guide (Appendix F) facilitate these steps.

- The appraisal process consists of determining the level of support for decision-making evidence and assessing the quality of that evidence to ensure it is adequate.

- The specific action items of the process will vary depending on the type of evidence the team is appraising.

- Pre-appraised evidence requires a suitability assessment and a quality assessment.

- Single studies with a formal study design require an assessment of the design to determine the level of support for decision-making, followed by a quality assessment.

- Anecdotal evidence requires a quality assessment.

OBJECTIVES

- 8.1 Describe the different paths EBP projects may take (understanding)

- 8.2 Differentiate between the different types of single-study evidence (analyzing)

- 8.3 Recognize evidence terminology and important considerations (understanding)

- 8.4 Appraise evidence using a guide (evaluating)

LEARNING ACTIVITIES

Before completion of the learning activities, you should do the following:

- Read Chapter 8
- Download the Appraisal Tool Selection Algorithm (Appendix D), Pre-Appraised Evidence Appraisal Tool (Appendix E1), Single Study Evidence Appraisal Tool (Appendix E2), Anecdotal Evidence Appraisal Tool (Appendix E3), and Evidence Terminology and Considerations Guide (Appendix F) (Hopkins.org/tools)
- Read Article 1: https://academic.oup.com/ageing/article/53/7/afae149/7716267
- Read Article 2: https://jamanetwork.com/journals/jamanetworkopen/fullarticle/2773051#google_vignette
- Read Article 3: https://www.the-hospitalist.org/hospitalist/article/36605/critical-care/how-can-hospitalists-help-reduce-harmful-in-hospital-patient-falls/

Learning Activity 8.1

Read the following summaries of five fictional articles. For each, use the Appraisal Tool Selection Algorithm (Appendix D; see Figure 8.1) to determine 1) the level of support for decision-making and 2) which appraisal tool best suits the evidence described.

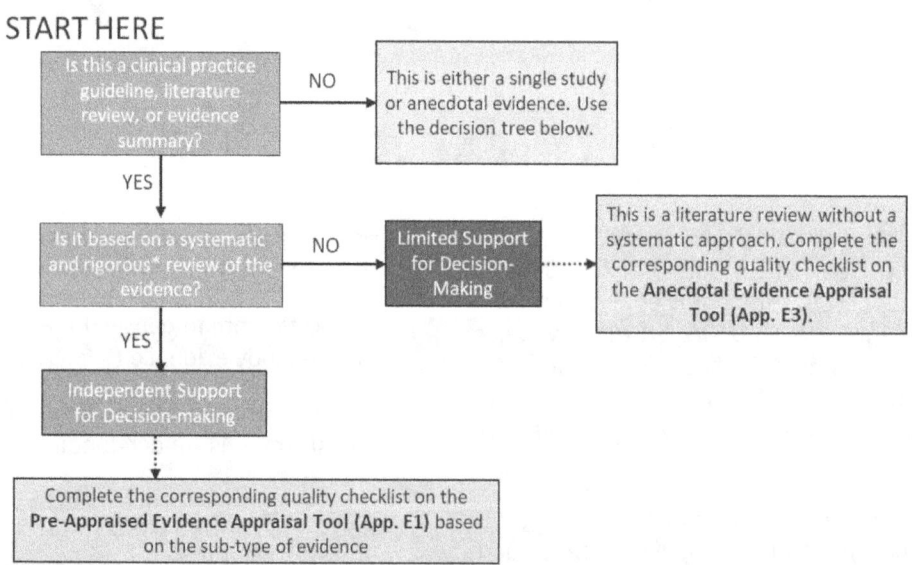

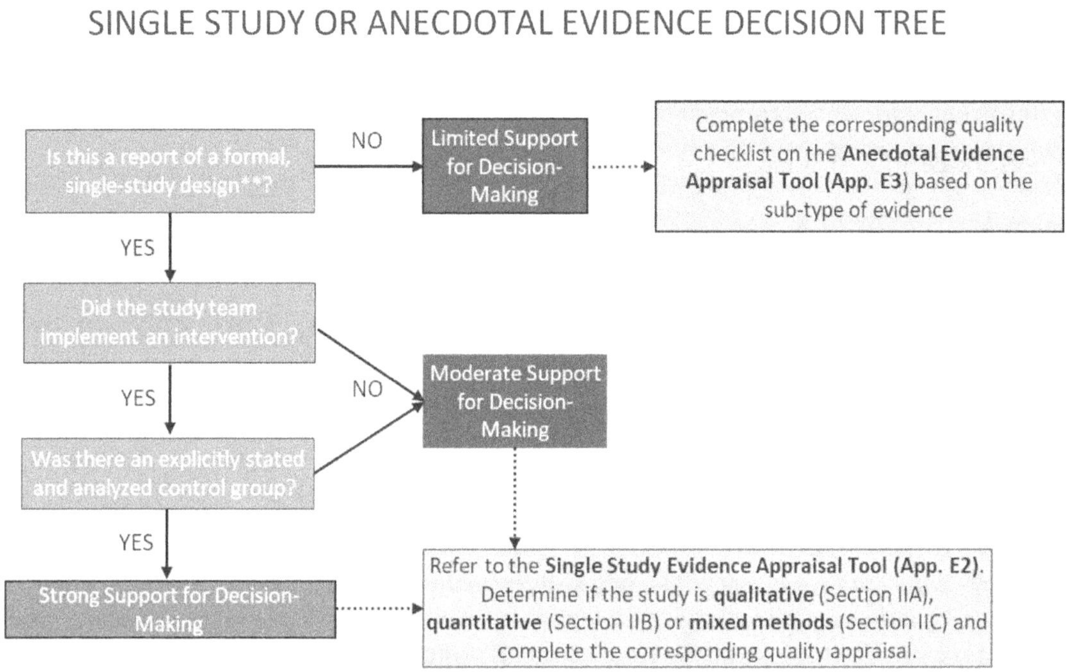

SINGLE STUDY OR ANECDOTAL EVIDENCE DECISION TREE

FIGURE 8.1 Appraisal Tool Selection Algorithm (Appendix D).

A systematic review with meta-analysis explores the use of artificial intelligence (AI) in healthcare. The authors all appear to be experts in the field of study. Twenty-five articles were included in the review, and definitive inclusion/exclusion criteria were established. The quality of the included studies was clearly established. The researchers reported following PRISMA guidelines to conduct the review.

Level of support for decision-making:

A. Independent   B. Strong   C. Moderate   D. Limited

Appraisal tool to consult:

A. Pre-appraised Evidence Appraisal Tool (Appendix E1)

B. Single Study Evidence Appraisal Tool (Appendix E2)

C. Anecdotal Evidence Appraisal Tool (Appendix E3)

A journal article provides a review of several studies on nurses' use of AI. The author explores what is known about the topic and provides a summary of the evidence. No formal process or protocol for the review was provided. Twelve references were included, though no analysis of their strengths or weaknesses is evident. The author concludes with recommendations for further study and implications for practice.

Level of support for decision-making:

    A. Independent   B. Strong   C. Moderate   D. Limited

Appraisal tool to consult:

    A. Pre-appraised Evidence Appraisal Tool (Appendix E1)

    B. Single Study Evidence Appraisal Tool (Appendix E2)

    C. Anecdotal Evidence Appraisal Tool (Appendix E3)

An article describes a research study using AI to determine the frequency of turning for ICU patients. The researchers reported a "quasi-experimental study design" that received approval from the ethical review board. The study team used an AI system to develop a turning protocol for all patients in the ICU. They monitored rates of pressure injury for six weeks following initiation of the protocol.

Level of support for decision-making:

    A. Independent   B. Strong   C. Moderate   D. Limited

Appraisal tool to consult:

    A. Pre-appraised Evidence Appraisal Tool (Appendix E1)

    B. Single Study Evidence Appraisal Tool (Appendix E2)

    C. Anecdotal Evidence Appraisal Tool (Appendix E3)

In a randomized control trial, researchers report receiving ethical review approval for a 12-week study of the impact of AI-generated patient teaching materials on patients' understanding of discharge instructions. Patients randomized into the intervention group received AI handouts tailored to their unique medical history. The other patients received generic materials generated from the electronic medical record. Patients were surveyed at discharge, at one month, and at three months using a validated instrument.

Level of support for decision-making:

    A. Independent   B. Strong   C. Moderate   D. Limited

Appraisal tool to consult:

    A. Pre-appraised Evidence Appraisal Tool (Appendix E1)

    B. Single Study Evidence Appraisal Tool (Appendix E2)

    C. Anecdotal Evidence Appraisal Tool (Appendix E3)

An article provides details of an organization's initiative aimed at decreasing the time it takes for medications to be received on the unit once an order has been placed. AI software was used to read and verify the orders for accuracy, check the patient's record for any contraindications, and ensure there is adequate hospital supply of the medication/dosage. A pharmacist would then double-check the results and send the order to be filled. Both the pharmacist and the unit staff reported improved efficiency.

Level of support for decision-making:

A. Independent   B. Strong   C. Moderate   D. Limited

Appraisal tool to consult:

A. Pre-appraised Evidence Appraisal Tool (Appendix E1)

B. Single Study Evidence Appraisal Tool (Appendix E2)

C. Anecdotal Evidence Appraisal Tool (Appendix E3)

Learning Activity 8.2

Differentiate the different types of single-study evidence. Complete the following table based on your readings.

FEATURE	RANDOMIZED CONTROL TRIAL	QUASI-EXPERIMENTAL	DESCRIPTIVE	QUALITATIVE
Type of study	Experimental			
Randomization			No	
Control group		May or may not have		
Purpose				
Data type	Quantitative			
Strengths				Rich, deep understanding of human experience
Limitations			Cannot establish causality; limited by bias	

Learning Activity 8.3

Part 1: Define bias and identify some considerations, including the relationship of quality assessment to bias.

	DEFINITION	CONSIDERATIONS
Bias		

Part 2: Using the definitions provided in the following table, identify the type of bias described in the five examples.

TYPES OF BIAS IN RESEARCH

Selection bias	Occurs when participants are not randomly selected, leading to a non-representative sample
Measurement bias	Occurs when the tools or methods used to measure variables are inaccurate or inconsistent
Observer bias	Occurs when the researcher's expectations or beliefs influence how they observe or record data
Recall bias	Occurs in self-reported data where participants may not accurately remember past events or experiences
Publication bias	Occurs when studies with positive or significant results are more likely to be published than those with null or negative findings
Performance bias	Occurs when there is a difference in how participants are treated in different groups, apart from the intervention being studied

1. Researchers developed a study to examine the effectiveness of a new drug. The sample only includes participants who volunteer to take part. These participants are more likely to be healthier and more motivated to follow the treatment protocol.

    Type of bias identified: _____

2. Researchers are investigating a new product to promote sleep in hospitalized patients. A retrospective study on sleep products asks participants to recall the quality of their sleep in past hospitalizations (within five years) and what sleep interventions were beneficial. Participants may not remember sleep disruptions or intervention used.

   Type of bias identified: _____

3. A professor studies two teaching methods but the students in one group are taught by a more experienced teacher, while the other group is taught by a less experienced teacher.

   Type of bias identified: _____

4. A sleep researcher only publishes studies where a treatment shows significant effects and not those studies where no effects were observed.

   Type of bias identified: _____

5. In a qualitative study, the researcher conducts interviews with participants to explore their experiences with cancer treatment. While transcribing the commentary, the researcher overlooks any reports of negative interactions with physicians believing the patients' reports must be mistaken.

   Type of bias identified: _____

Learning Activity 8.4

Part 1: Read the following case study excerpt.

With your newly formed EBP team, you conduct a best-evidence search of the literature. Your team finds a pre-appraised article that answers the EBP question.

After considering the information in the case study excerpt, read and appraise article 1 and complete the Pre-appraised Evidence Appraisal Tool (Appendix E1; see Figure 8.2).

Article 1: https://academic.oup.com/ageing/article/53/7/afae149/7716267

Pre-Appraised Evidence Appraisal Tool

Fill in this data collection table after completing the suitability and quality assessments below.						
Article Number	Author, date, title	Type of pre-appraised evidence	Topic or intervention	Population	Setting	Recommendations that answer the EBP question

*For definitions of terms in **bold print** see **Appendix F: Evidence Terminology and Considerations Guide**

Section I: Suitability

Only complete this section if you are using this evidence as potential independent support for decision-making. **If you gathered this evidence in an exhaustive search, skip to Section II: Quality Appraisal.**

	Yes	No	Unclear	N/A
Is the topic or intervention the same or similar to the topic of interest?				
Is the population the same or similar to your population of interest?				
Is the setting the same or similar to your setting of interest?				
If applicable, are the **outcomes** the same or similar to your **outcomes** of interest?				
How recent are the references (*provide date*)?				
Are the references recent enough to be reasonably applied to the practice setting (this will depend on the intervention and changing nature of the topic at hand)				
Notes:				

*For independent support for decision-making, all responses must be YES. If the topic, population, setting, or outcome is similar, but not the same, include in the notes section the team's rationale for how the provided information can be reasonably compared to the elements in the team's EBP question. **If suitable, complete the corresponding quality assessment below.**

If the evidence is not fully suitable, but it informs the EBP question, complete the appraisal below. If the quality is adequate, this is strong support for decision-making, record the information on Appendix G2: The Individual Evidence Summary Tool.

Section II: Quality Appraisal

Complete the checklist below for the corresponding sub-type of evidence.

Evidence Summary (point-of-care clinical decision support produced by a reputable organization)

	Yes	No	Unclear	N/A
1. Was the summary produced by a reputable organization?				
2. Does the organization use a clear, systematic, and comprehensive method for selecting evidence?**				
3. Does the organization use a clear, well-established process for evaluating evidence (e.g. rapid review protocol, systematic review)?**				
4. Is the **review question** or summary topic clearly stated?				
5. Are the details of the included evidence provided (including types of studies, intervention(s), settings, populations, and **grading**)?				
6. Is there a direct and obvious link between recommendations and the provided evidence?				
7. Are recommendations clear and complete (including a **level of certainty/confidence**)?				
8. Does the **level of certainty/confidence** of each of the recommendations align with the evidence used to support them?				
9. Did the review undergo an independent peer review?				
10. Are funding and **conflicts of interest** addressed?				

** This may be directly provided or available on the organization's website

Consider all of your responses above. Do you think the quality of this article is adequate to provide independent support for decision-making?

☐ Yes → *Include, complete data collection table on page 1*
☐ No → *Exclude, set aside, and note exclusion for tracking*

Clinical Practice Guidelines

	Yes	No	Unclear	N/A
1. Is the review group made up of experts who have proven expertise or skills related to the topic?				
2. Is the target population of the recommendations clear?				
3. Is the process for making the recommendations provided (e.g. evidence review, reaching consensus)?				
4. Are recommendations clear and complete (including a level of certainty/confidence)?				

	Yes	No	Unclear	N/A
5. Was there an external, peer-review of the guidelines?				

8 EVIDENCE PHASE: APPRAISING THE EVIDENCE 71

6. Does the level of certainty/confidence of each of the recommendations align with the evidence used to support them?				
7. Are funding and conflicts of interest addressed?				
Complete the below checklist to determine the quality of the literature review used to generate the guidelines.				
Literature Reviews with a Systematic Approach (LRSAs)				
	Yes	No	Unclear	N/A
Background/Introduction				
1. Is a logical background and rationale for the review explained regarding current literature?				
2. Is the review question clear?				
Methods				
1. Did the review follow a model or guideline (e.g. PRISMA, AMSTAR II, etc.)?				
2. Do the authors clearly state what they are trying to measure or describe?				
3. Was the literature search thorough and could it be replicated (this includes providing keywords, inclusion/exclusion criteria, and at least 2 formal databases searched)?				
4. Was there an independent double-check system in the review process (this includes an independent assessment for eligibility, critical appraisal, and data extraction by at least 2 reviewers for each article)?				
5. Was the quality of each included study formally assessed and listed?				
6. Was the risk of introducing bias into the literature selection and review process addressed and minimized?				
7. If applicable, were data pooling (meta-analysis or meta-synthesis) methods clear and appropriate?				
8. In addition to the items above, did the authors answer all of your questions about how they conducted their review [include notes about additional concerns]?				
Results				
1. Was there a flow diagram that included the number of studies eliminated at each stage of the review?				
2. Were details of included studies provided (e.g. design, sample, methods, results, outcomes, limitations, the strength of evidence)?				
3. If applicable, are themes identified?				
4. If applicable, are statistics shown clearly?				
	Yes	No	Unclear	N/A
Discussion				
1. Does the discussion match what is reported in the results section?				
2. Do the authors examine what they found and compare it to other literature on the topic?				
3. Are limitations included with an explanation of how they were handled?				
4. Do the authors provide implications of their study for practice and future investigation?				
General				
1. Is all the information in the paper congruent (consistent throughout the aims, methods, results, and discussion sections)?				
2. Are funding and conflict(s) of interest addressed?				
Consider all of your responses above. Do you think the quality of this article is adequate to provide independent support for decision-making?	☐ Yes → *Include, complete data collection table on page 1* ☐ No → *Exclude, set aside, and note exclusion for tracking*			

FIGURE 8.2 Pre-appraised Evidence Appraisal Tool (Appendix E1).

Part 2: Read the following case study excerpt.

Now suppose, after a best-evidence search of the literature, your team did not find a pre-appraised article that answers the EBP question. Your team moves forward with an exhaustive literature search. Your team finds a total of 84 articles that answer the EBP question, including both single studies and anecdotal evidence.

After considering the information in the case study excerpt, use the Appraisal Tool Selection Algorithm (Appendix D, refer to Figure 8.1) to determine the level of support for decision-making and the appropriate appraisal tool to use to appraise Articles 2 and 3 and mark your answers on the following chart.

Article 2: https://jamanetwork.com/journals/jamanetworkopen/fullarticle/2773051#google_ vignette

Article 3: https://www.the-hospitalist.org/hospitalist/article/36605/critical-care/how-can-hospitalists-help-reduce-harmful-in-hospital-patient-falls/

ARTICLE #	ARTICLE OVERVIEW	LEVEL OF SUPPORT FOR DECISION-MAKING	EVIDENCE APPRAISAL TOOL
2			
3			

Part 3: Appraise Articles 2 and 3 using the appropriate evidence appraisal tools. Fill out one appraisal tool for each article (see Figures 8.3 and 8.4).

Single Study Evidence Appraisal Tool

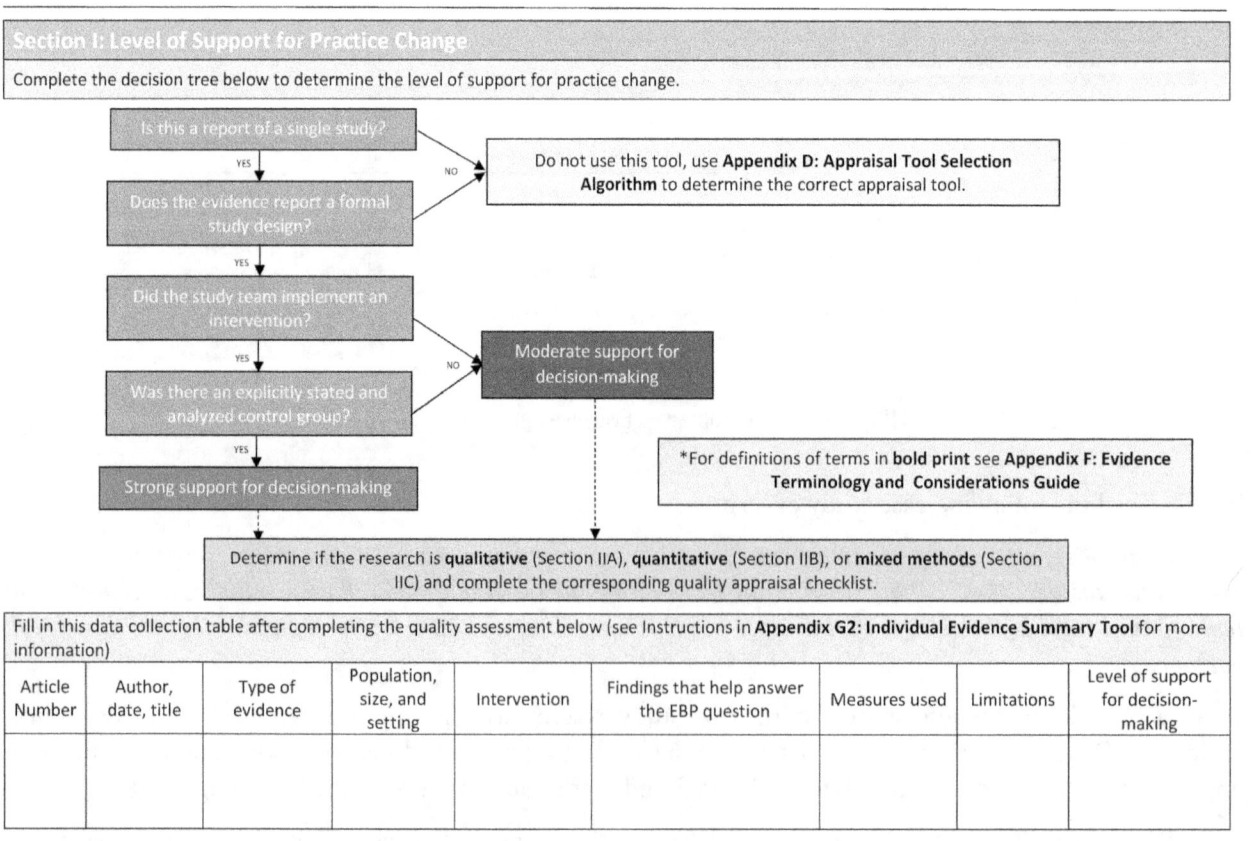

© 2025 Johns Hopkins Health System

Section II: Quality Appraisal

Complete the checklist below for the corresponding type of evidence.

Section IIA: Qualitative Evidence

	Yes	No	Unclear	N/A
Introduction/Background				
1. Is a logical background and rationale for the study explained using **current** literature?				
2. Is the purpose/objective of the study clear?				
Methods				
1. Is the **study design** and guiding theory or model provided with the reason it was chosen?				
2. Is the **study setting** clearly described (including location, dates, and other important details) to enhance **transferability**?				
3. Is the process for recruiting participants (**sampling**) explained clearly and does it match with the study aim(s)?				
4. Do **eligibility** criteria (rules for who can join the study) make sense and are they easy to understand?				
5. Is the **sample size** adequate, as shown by reaching data **saturation**?				
6. Are important characteristics of the group they studied (**sample**) provided (e.g. how many participants or encounters were involved, demographics, or other details about the participants or things being studied)?				
7. Did the authors address **reflexivity** (how their background or experience might have affected the study)?				
8. Are the **data collection** methods clear and appropriate (this includes how they gathered and recorded the information)?				
9. Are **data processing** methods clear and appropriate (this includes how the data was transcribed and checked) to enhance **credibility**?				
10. Are the methods to **analyze** the data well explained (this includes what computer programs they used and how they coded the data to find patterns or themes) to enhance **confirmability**?				
11. Are the **intervention**(s) clearly described?				
12. Is there information on the **ethical review** provided?				
13. In addition to the items above, did the authors answer all of your questions about how they conducted their study (include notes about additional concerns)?				
Results/Findings				
1. Do the findings make sense and are they easy to understand?				

	Yes	No	Unclear	N/A
2. Are **themes or patterns** identified clearly?				
3. Do the authors provide enough quotations, detailed observations, or other proof to support their findings?				
Discussion				
1. Does the discussion match what is reported in the results section?				
2. Do the authors examine what they found and compare it to other literature on the topic?				
3. Are **limitations** included with an explanation of how they were handled?				
4. Do the authors provide implications of their study for practice and future investigation?				
General				
1. Is all the information in the paper **congruent** (consistent throughout the aims, methods, results, and discussion sections)?				
2. Are funding and **conflicts of interest** addressed?				

Consider all of your responses above. Do you think the quality of this article is adequate to provide dependable information to answer your EBP question?	☐ Yes → *Include, complete data collection table on page 1* ☐ No → *Exclude, set aside, and note exclusion for tracking*

Section IIB: Quantitative Evidence

	Yes	No	Unclear	N/A
Introduction/Background				
1. Is a logical background and rationale for the study explained using **current** literature?				
2. Is the purpose/objective of the study clear?				
Methods				
1. Is the **study design** clearly stated?				
2. Is the **study setting** clearly described (including location, dates, and other important details) to enhance **generalizability**?				
3. Is the process for recruiting participants (**sampling**) explained clearly and does it match with the study aim(s)?				
4. Do **eligibility** criteria (rules for who can join the study) make sense and are they easy to understand?				
5. Is the **sample size powered** adequately (a calculation or other explanation for how the authors decided how many participants or observations to include)?				
6. Did the authors clearly state what they wanted to measure?				

	Yes	No	Unclear	N/A
7. Are the **data collection** methods clear and appropriate (this includes how they gathered and recorded the information)?				

continues

(cont'd)

	Yes	No	Unclear	N/A
a) If applicable, were all the tools **reliable**?				
b) If applicable, were all the tools **valid**?				
8. Are the methods to analyze the data well explained (this includes what computer programs they used, how they made calculations or anything else they did to explore the data)?				
9. If applicable, are the intervention(s) clearly described?				
10. If there was **randomization**,				
a) Was true **randomization** used to put people in the **control** and **intervention** groups?				
b) Other than the intervention being studied, were the **intervention** and **control** groups treated similarly?				
11. Is there information on the **ethical review** provided?				
12. In addition to the items above, did the authors answer all of your questions about how they conducted their study [include notes about additional concerns]?				
Results/Findings				
1. Do the findings make sense and are they easy to understand?				
2. Are characteristics of the participants provided (this may include demographics or other important details about the participants or things being studied)?				
3. If applicable, was the survey **response rate** provided?				
4. If applicable, are **attrition** rates provided (this includes how many people remained with the study at each stage)?				
5. Is data provided for each item the authors stated they wanted to measure?				
6. If applicable, are the baseline characteristics of the **intervention** and **control** groups similar?				
7. Are any statistics shown clearly?				
Discussion				
1. Does the discussion match what is reported in the results section?				
2. Do the authors examine what they found and compare it to other literature on the topic?				
3. Are **limitations** included with an explanation of how they were handled?				
4. Do the authors provide implications of their study for practice and future investigation?				

	Yes	No	Unclear	N/A
General				
1. Is all the information in the paper **congruent** (consistent throughout the aims, methods, results, and discussion sections)?				
2. Are funding and **conflicts of interest** addressed?				
Consider all of your responses above. Do you think the quality of this article is adequate to provide dependable information to answer your EBP question?	☐ Yes → *Include, complete data collection table on page 1* ☐ No → *Exclude, set aside, and note exclusion for tracking*			

Section IIC: Mixed Methods Evidence

	Yes	No	Unclear	N/A
Background/Introduction				
1. Is a logical background and rationale for the review explained regarding **current** literature?				
2. Is the purpose/objective of the study clear?				
Methods				
1. Is the **study design** and mixed methods approach clearly stated with an explanation of why it was chosen?				
2. Is the **study setting** clearly described (including location, dates, and other important details) to enhance **generalizability**?				
3. Is the process for recruiting participants (**sampling**) explained clearly and does it match with the study aim(s)?				
4. Do **eligibility** criteria (rules for who can join the study) make sense and are they easy to understand?				
5. Is the **sample size** adequate…				
a) For the qualitative portion (this includes evidence of data saturation)?				
b) For the quantitative portion (this includes adequate **power**, a calculation, or other explanation for how the authors decided how many participants or observations to include)?				
6. Did the authors clearly state what they wanted to measure or describe?				
7. Did the authors address **reflexivity** (how their background or experience might have affected the study)?				
8. If applicable, are the **intervention**(s) clearly described?				
9. Are the **data collection** methods clear and appropriate (this includes how they gathered and recorded the information)?				
a) If applicable, were all the tools **reliable**?				
	Yes	No	Unclear	N/A

b) If applicable, were all the tools **valid**?				
10. In the qualitative section, are data processing methods clear and appropriate (this includes how the data was transcribed and checked) to enhance **credibility**?				
11. Are the methods to **analyze** the data well explained...				
a) For the qualitative section (this includes coding and generation of themes)?				
b) For the quantitative section (this includes what computer programs they used, how they made calculations, or anything else they did to explore the data)?				
12. If there was **randomization**,				
a) Was true **randomization** used to put people in the **control** and **intervention** groups?				
b) Other than the intervention being studied, were the **intervention** and **control** groups treated similarly?				
13. Do the authors truly use and integrate both qualitative and quantitative methodologies to collect and analyze data?				
14. Is there information on the **ethical review** provided?				
15. In addition to the items above, did the authors answer all of your questions about how they conducted their study? [include notes about additional concerns]				
Results				
1. Do the **findings** make sense and are they easy to understand?				
2. Are characteristics of the participants provided (this may include demographics or other important details about the participants or things being studied)?				
3. If applicable, was the survey **response rate** provided?				
4. If applicable, are **attrition** rates provided (this includes how many people remained with the study at each stage)?				
5. Is data provided for each item the authors stated they wanted to measure or describe?				
6. In the qualitative section, do the authors provide enough quotations, detailed observations, or other proof to support their findings?				
7. In the quantitative section, are statistics shown clearly?				
8. If applicable, are the baseline characteristics of the **intervention** and **control** groups similar?				
9. Are any statistics shown clearly?				

	Yes	No	Unclear	N/A
Discussion				
1. Does the discussion match what is reported in the results section?				
2. Do the authors fully integrate the qualitative and quantitative data to create a deeper understanding?				
3. Do the authors examine what they found and compare it to other literature on the topic?				
4. Are **limitations** included with an explanation of how they were handled?				
5. Do the authors provide implications of their study for practice and future investigation?				
General				
1. Is all the information in the paper **congruent** (consistent throughout the aims, methods, results, and discussion sections)?				
2. Are funding and **conflicts of interest** addressed?				
Consider all of your responses above. Do you think the quality of this article is adequate to provide dependable information to answer your EBP question?	☐ Yes → *Include, complete data collection table on page 1* ☐ No → *Exclude, set aside, and note exclusion for tracking*			

FIGURE 8.3 Single Study Evidence Appraisal Tool (Appendix E2).

Anecdotal Evidence Appraisal Tool

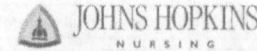

Fill in this data collection table after completing the quality assessment below (see Instructions in **Appendix G2: Individual Evidence Summary Tool** for more information).

Article Number	Author, date, title	Type of evidence	Population, size, and setting	Intervention	Findings that help answer the EBP question	Measures used	Limitations	Level of support for decision-making?
								Limited

*For definitions of terms in **bold print** see **Appendix F: Evidence Terminology and Considerations Guide**

Section I: Quality Appraisal

Complete the checklist below for the corresponding sub-type of evidence. Note, the headers within each checklist are used for organization and may not match the exact language from the article or report being appraised

Expert Opinion, Position Statements, and Book Chapters				
	Yes	No	Unclear	N/A
Author(s) expertise				
1. Does the author(s) know about the topic of interest as evidenced by previous publications on the topic, relevant professional or academic **affiliations**, related education/training, or other activities that suggest their **expertise**?				
Purpose/objectives				
1. Is the purpose/objective(s) clearly stated?				
Reference to evidence				
1. Is there a thorough reference to **current** literature on the topic?				
2. Do the author(s) provide meaningful **analysis** (through insights or commentary) of existing evidence on the topic?				
Summary/conclusions				
1. Is it clear and logical how the authors reached their conclusion(s)?				
2. Are recommendations clear?				
	Yes	No	Unclear	N/A
General				
1. Are funding and **conflicts of interest** addressed?				

Consider all of your responses above. Do you think the quality of this article is adequate to provide dependable information to answer your EBP question?
- ☐ Yes → Include, complete data collection table on page 1
- ☐ No → Exclude, set aside, and note exclusion for tracking

Case Report				
	Yes	No	Unclear	N/A
Introduction				
1. Is there a short introduction to the case, including why it is relevant or important?				
Patient information				
1. Is patient-level data provided to address the clinical focus of the case study (this can include patient history, clinical findings, diagnosis, or timeline)?				
2. Is there a thorough explanation of diagnostic and/or therapeutic intervention(s)?				
3. Did the patient or caregiver provide informed consent?				
Discussion				
1. Is their meaningful interpretation of the patient information (see above)?				
2. Are "lessons learned" clearly stated and based on the provided patient information?				
3. Is there an insightful discussion of the case presentation regarding relevant medical literature?				
General				
1. Are funding and **conflicts of interest** addressed?				
2. Is the information provided in a logical manner that is easy to follow?				

Consider all of your responses above. Do you think the quality of this article is adequate to provide dependable information to answer your EBP question?
- ☐ Yes → Include, complete data collection table on page 1
- ☐ No → Exclude, set aside, and note exclusion for tracking

Programmatic Experiences				
	Yes	No	Unclear	N/A
Introduction				

	Yes	No	Unclear	N/A
1. Is there a short introduction to the project, including why it is relevant or important?				
2. Is the purpose/objective of the project clear?				
Project Information				
1. Is there adequate information regarding the context of the project, including the setting and people involved?				
2. Is what the project team did (interventions) clearly described?				
3. Was a tool, model, or framework used to plan and implement the project?				
4. Are the findings or impact of the project provided?				
Discussion				
1. Does the author(s) provide insights into the project's successes and areas for improvement?				
2. Are "lessons learned" clearly stated?				
3. Is the project discussed in the context of **currently** available information on the intervention or problem it was addressing?				
General				
1. Are funding and **conflicts of interest** addressed?				
2. Are you able to follow what the group did to implement and measure the success of the project?				
Consider all of your responses above. Do you think the quality of this article is adequate to provide dependable information to answer your EBP question?	☐ Yes → *Include, complete data collection table on page 1* ☐ No → *Exclude, set aside, and note exclusion for tracking*			

Reviews with an Unsystematic Approach (e.g., Scoping, Critical, Literature Reviews)

	Yes	No	Unclear	N/A
Background/Introduction				
1. Is a logical background and rationale for the review explained regarding current literature?				
2. Is the review question clear?				
Methods				
1. Did the review follow a model or guideline?				
2. Do the authors clearly state what they are trying to measure or describe?				
3. Do the authors explain how they selected the articles included in their review?				

© 2025 Johns Hopkins Health System

Results				
1. Are findings from the included articles presented clearly?				
Discussion				
1. Does the discussion match what is reported in the results section?				
2. Is it clear how the authors arrived at their conclusions?				
General				
1. Are funding and **conflicts of interest** addressed?				
Consider all of your responses above. Do you think the quality of this article is adequate to provide dependable information to answer your EBP question?	☐ Yes → *Include, complete data collection table on page 1* ☐ No → *Exclude, set aside, and note exclusion for tracking*			

FIGURE 8.4 Anecdotal Evidence Appraisal Tool (Appendix E3).

CALL TO ACTION

It is time to appraise the evidence gathered from your search (either best-evidence or exhaustive). Use the Appraisal Tool Selection Algorithm (Appendix D) to determine 1) the level of support for decision-making and 2) which appraisal tool best suits the evidence at hand.

Appraise each piece of evidence using the appropriate tool, noting the level of support for decision-making and overall quality. Refer to the Evidence Terminology and Considerations Guide (Appendix F) to learn about new or unfamiliar terms as well as what to consider when appraising.

If you are unable to find any suitable evidence to answer the EBP question, you cannot move further with the project. Consider adjusting the search terms, reevaluating the question, or further clarifying the problem. If no evidence exists, teams can wait for more evidence to be published, continue with current practice, and/or conduct a research study to answer the question.

DISCUSSION QUESTIONS

1. What is the purpose of the appraisal process in EBP, and how does it contribute to the overall quality of the team's decision-making?
2. How should an EBP team approach the appraisal of different types of evidence, and what special considerations are necessary for each type?
3. What criteria can be used to assess the relevance, validity, and reliability of evidence during the appraisal process, and why are these criteria important for ensuring high-quality recommendations?
4. How does a well-conducted appraisal process prepare an EBP team for the steps of summarizing, synthesizing, and generating best-evidence recommendations? What are the potential risks of advancing without thorough appraisal?
5. Reflect on a time when evidence was appraised incorrectly or insufficiently. What impact might this have on patient care, and how can EBP teams avoid similar pitfalls in their appraisal process?

A CLOSER LOOK

The Johns Hopkins EBP Appraisal Tools (Appendices E1, E2, and E3)

To appraise the evidence, use the Pre-appraised Evidence Appraisal Tool, Single Study Evidence Appraisal Tool, and Anecdotal Evidence Appraisal Tool (see Figures 8.5, 8.6, and 8.7).

Pre-Appraised Evidence Appraisal Tool

Fill in this data collection table after completing the suitability and quality assessments below.

Article Number	Author, date, title	Type of pre-appraised evidence	Topic or intervention	Population	Setting	Recommendations that answer the EBP question

> Numbering articles as they are reviewed helps to keep the evidence organized.

*For definitions of terms in **bold print** see **Appendix F: Evidence Terminology and Considerations Guide**

Section I: Suitability

Only complete this section if you are using this evidence as potential independent support for decision-making. **If you gathered this evidence in an exhaustive search, skip to Section II: Quality Appraisal.**

	Yes	No	Unclear	N/A
Is the topic or intervention the same or similar to the topic of interest?				
Is the population the same or similar to your population of interest?				
Is the setting the same or similar to your setting of interest?				
If applicable, are the **outcomes** the same or similar to your **outcomes** of interest?				
How recent are the references (*provide date*)?				
Are the references recent enough to be reasonably applied to the practice setting (this will depend on the intervention and changing nature of the topic at hand)				

Notes:

> All bolded terms are defined in the Evidence Terminology and Considerations Guide (Appendix F).

*For independent support for decision-making, all responses must be YES. If the topic, population, setting, or outcome is similar, but not the same, include in the notes section the team's rationale for how the provided information can be reasonably compared to the elements in the team's EBP question. **If suitable, complete the corresponding quality assessment below.**

If the evidence is not fully suitable, but it informs the EBP question, complete the appraisal below. If the quality is adequate, this is strong support for decision-making, record the information on Appendix G2: The Individual Evidence Summary Tool.

Section II: Quality Appraisal

Complete the checklist below for the corresponding sub-type of evidence.

Evidence Summary (point-of-care clinical decision support produced by a reputable organization)

	Yes	No	Unclear	N/A
1. Was the summary produced by a reputable organization?				
2. Does the organization use a clear, systematic, and comprehensive method for selecting evidence?**				
3. Does the organization use a clear, well-established process for evaluating evidence (e.g. rapid review protocol, systematic review)?**				
4. Is the **review question** or summary topic clearly stated?				
5. Are the details of the included evidence provided (including types of studies, intervention(s), settings, populations, and **grading**)?				
6. Is there a direct and obvious link between recommendations and the provided evidence?				
7. Are recommendations clear and complete (including a **level of certainty/confidence**)?				
8. Does the **level of certainty/confidence** of each of the recommendations align with the evidence used to support them?				
9. Did the review undergo an independent peer review?				
10. Are funding and **conflicts of interest** addressed?				

** This may be directly provided or available on the organization's website

> There are sections for appraisal of each type of pre-appraised evidence. Make sure you are using the correct section.

Consider all of your responses above. Do you think the quality of this article is adequate to provide independent support for decision-making?

☐ Yes → *Include, complete data collection table on page 1*
☐ No → *Exclude, set aside, and note exclusion for tracking*

Clinical Practice Guidelines

	Yes	No	Unclear	N/A
1. Is the review group made up of experts...				
2. Is the target population of the recom...				
3. Is the process for making the recom...				
4. Are recommendations clear and co...				
5. Was there an external, peer-review of the guidelines?				

> After appraising the evidence, teams simply need to determine if the quality is good enough for independent decision-making.

FIGURE 8.5 Pre-appraised Evidence Appraisal Tool (Appendix E1), annotated.

Single Study Evidence Appraisal Tool

Section I: Level of Support for Practice Change

Complete the decision tree below to determine the level of support for practice change.

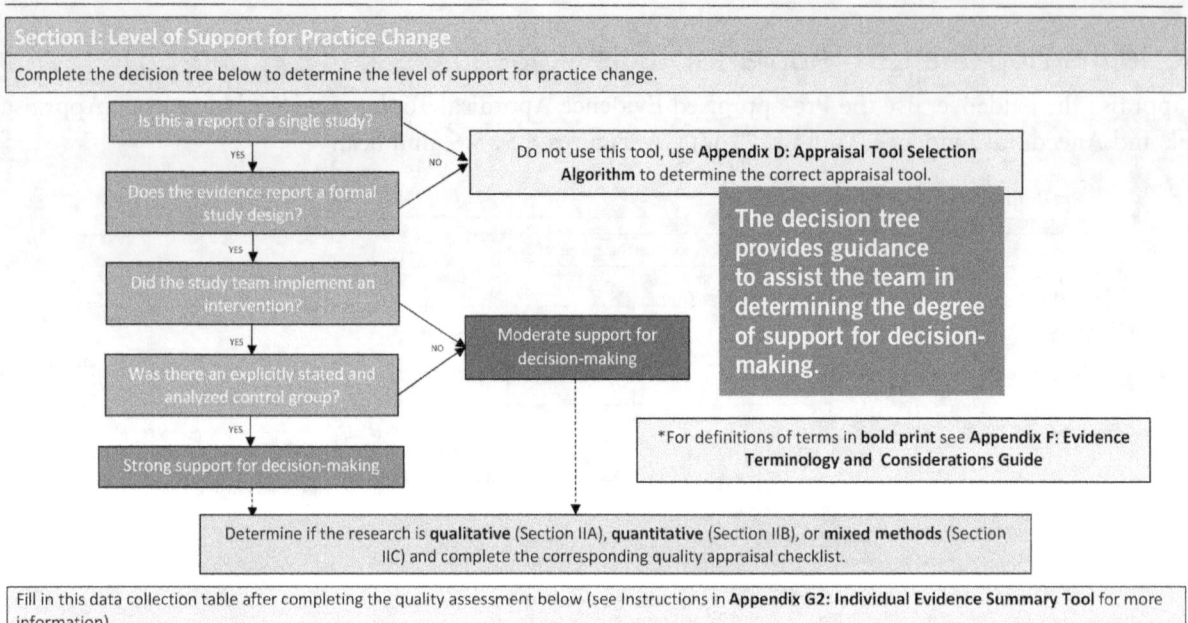

*For definitions of terms in **bold** print see **Appendix F: Evidence Terminology and Considerations Guide**

Determine if the research is **qualitative** (Section IIA), **quantitative** (Section IIB), or **mixed methods** (Section IIC) and complete the corresponding quality appraisal checklist.

Fill in this data collection table after completing the quality assessment below (see Instructions in **Appendix G2: Individual Evidence Summary Tool** for more information)

Article Number	Author, date, title	Type of evidence	Population, size, and setting	Intervention	Findings that help answer the EBP question	Measures used	Limitations	Level of support for decision-making

Findings should be accurately presented as succinct statements that answer the EBP question.

Section II: Quality Appraisal

Complete the checklist below for the corresponding type of evidence.

Section IIA: Qualitative Evidence

	Yes	No	Unclear	N/A
Introduction/Background				
1. Is a logical background and rationale for the study explained using **current** literature?				
2. Is the purpose/objective of the study clear?				
Methods				
1. Is the **study design** and guiding theory or model provided with the reason it was chosen?				
2. Is the **study setting** clearly described (including location, dates, and other important details) to enhance **transferability**?				
3. Is the process for recruiting participants (**sampling**) explained clearly and does it match with the study aim(s)?				
4. Do **eligibility** criteria (rules for who can join the study) make sense and are they easy to understand?				
5. Is the **sample size** adequate, as shown by reaching data **saturation**?				
6. Are important characteristics of the group they studied (**sample**) provided (e.g. how many participants or encounters were involved, demographics, or other details about the participants or things being studied)?				
7. Did the authors address **reflexivity** (how their background or experience might have affected the study)?				
8. Are the **data collection** methods clear and appropriate (this includes how they gathered and recorded the information)?				
9. Are **data processing** methods clear and appropriate (this includes how the data was transcribed and checked) to enhance **credibility**?				
10. Are the methods to **analyze** the data well explained (this includes what computer programs they used and how they coded the data to find patterns or themes) to enhance **confirmability**?				
11. Are the **intervention**(s) clearly described?				
12. Is there information on the **ethical review** provided?				
13. In addition to the items above, did the authors answer all of your questions about how they conducted their study [include notes about additional concerns]?				
Results/Findings				
1. Do the findings make sense and are they easy to understand?				
	Yes	No	Unclear	N/A

The team should use the Quality Appraisal section that matches the evidence at hand.

2. Are **themes or patterns** identified clearly?				
3. Do the authors provide enough quotations, detailed observations, or other proof to support their findings?				
Discussion				
1. Does the discussion match what is reported in the results section?				
2. Do the authors examine what they found and compare it to other literature on the topic?				
3. Are **limitations** included with an explanation of how they were handled?				
4. Do the authors provide implications of their study for practice and future investigation?				
General				
1. Is all the information in the paper **congruent** (consistent throughout the aims, methods, results, and discussion sections)?				
2. Are funding and **conflicts of interest** addressed?				
Consider all of your responses above. Do you think the quality of this article is adequate to provide dependable information to answer your EBP question?	☐ Yes → *Include, complete data collection table on page 1* ☐ No → *Exclude, set aside, and note exclusion for tracking*			

Section IIB: Quantitative Evidence				
	Yes	No	Unclear	N/A
Introduction/Background				
1. Is a logical background and rationale for the study ...				
2. Is the purpose/objective of the study clear?				
Methods				
1. Is the **study design** clearly stated?				
2. Is the **study setting** clearly described (including loc...) to enhance generalizability?				
3. Is the process for recruiting participants (**sampling**) ... h the study aim(s)?				
4. Do **eligibility** criteria (rules for who can join the stu... derstand?				
5. Is the **sample size powered** adequately (a calculati... ors decided how many participants or observations to include)?				
6. Did the authors clearly state what they wanted to measure?				
	Yes	No	Unclear	N/A

> After completing the appraisal, the team must decide if the quality of the article provides dependable information or not. Articles providing dependable information move forward. Those deemed undependable are excluded.

FIGURE 8.6 Single Study Evidence Appraisal Tool (Appendix E2), annotated.

Anecdotal Evidence Appraisal Tool

> Anecdotal evidence always provides limited support for decision-making.

JOHNS HOPKINS NURSING

Fill in this data collection table after completing the quality assessment below (see Instructions in **Appendix G2: Individual Evidence Summary Tool** for more information).

Article Number	Author, date, title	Type of evidence	Population, size, and setting	Intervention	Findings that help answer the EBP question	Measures used	Limitations	Level of support for decision-making?
								Limited

*For definitions of terms in **bold print** see Appendix F: Evidence Terminology and Considerations Guide

Section I: Quality Appraisal

Complete the checklist below for the corresponding sub-type of evidence. Note, the headers within each checklist are used for organization and may not match the exact language from the article or report being appraised

Expert Opinion, Position Statements, and Book Chapters

	Yes	No	Unclear	N/A
Author(s) expertise				
1. Does the author(s) know about the topic of interest as evidenced by previous publications on the topic, relevant professional or academic **affiliations**, related education/training, or other activities that suggest their **expertise**?				
Purpose/objectives				
1. Is the purpose/objective(s) clearly stated?				
Reference to evidence				
1. Is there a...				
2. Do the au...				
Summary/con...				
1. Is it clear...				
2. Are recommendations clear?				

> As with other appraisal tools, there are different sections for the different types of anecdotal evidence. Ensure the section matches the type of evidence you have.

	Yes	No	Unclear	N/A
General				
1. Are funding and **conflicts of interest** addressed?				
Consider all of your responses above. Do you think the quality of this article is adequate to provide dependable information to answer your EBP question?	☐ Yes → *Include, complete data collection table on page 1* ☐ No → *Exclude, set aside, and note exclusion for tracking*			

Case Report

	Yes	No	Unclear	N/A
Introduction				
1. Is there a short introduction to the case, including why it is relevant or important?				
Patient information				
1. Is patient-level data provided to address the clinical focus of the case study (this can include patient history, clinical findings, diagnosis, or timeline)?				
2. Is there a thorough explanation of diagnostic and/or therapeutic intervention(s)?				
3. Did the patient or caregiver provide informed consent?				
Discussion				
1. Is their meaningful interpretation of the patient information (see above)?				
2. Are "lessons learned" clearly stated and based on the provided patient information?				
3. Is there an insightful discussion of the case presentation regarding relevant medical literature?				
General				
1. Are funding and **conflicts of interest** addressed?				
2. Is the information provided in a logical manner that is easy to follow?				
Consider all of your responses above. Do you think the quality of this article is adequate to provide dependable information to answer your EBP question?	☐ Yes → *Include, complete data collection table on page 1* ☐ No → *Exclude, set aside, and note exclusion for tracking*			

Programmatic Experiences

	Yes	No	Unclear	N/A
Introduction				

FIGURE 8.7 Anecdotal Evidence Appraisal Tool (Appendix E3), annotated.

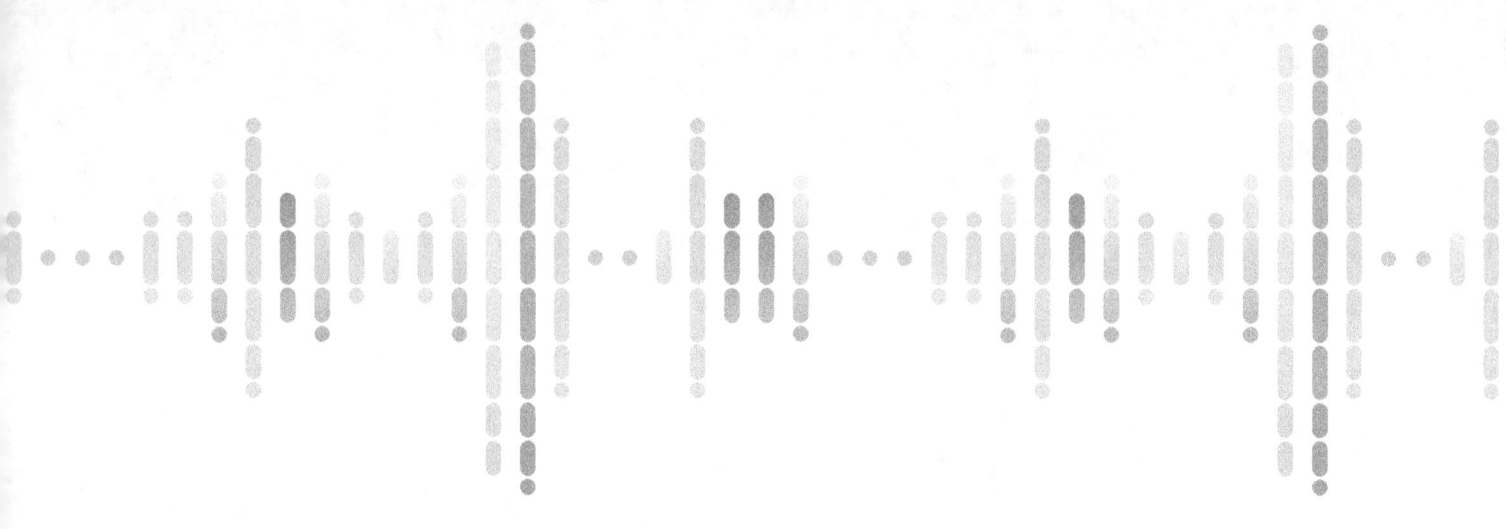

OVERVIEW

The evidence portion of the EBP project is the crux of the EBP process. Without an in-depth understanding of the evidence related to the practice problem, organizational change can at best falter and at worst cause harm. Best-evidence recommendations based on a robust synthesis with careful consideration and highly developed critical thinking can make a good EBP project a great one. This builds a strong and reliable foundation for organizational translation, which builds on the process with the addition of organizational context, including patient and provider preference.

9

EVIDENCE PHASE: SUMMARY, SYNTHESIS, AND BEST-EVIDENCE RECOMMENDATIONS

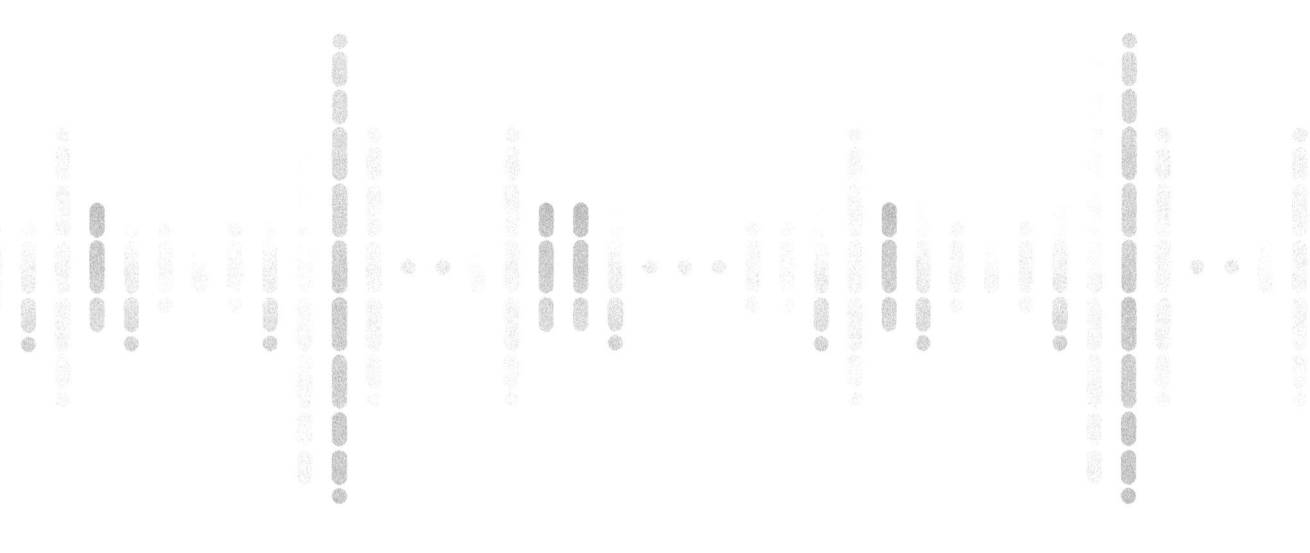

KEY POINTS

The evidence phase contains seven steps. This chapter provides an overview of Steps 7–10.

The JHEBP Best-Evidence Summary Tool (Appendix G1), Individual Evidence Summary Tool (Appendix G2), and Summary, Synthesis, & Best-Evidence Recommendations Tool (Appendix H) facilitate these steps.

- *Evidence summary* is the process of collating essential information from articles or reports into a central location. The EBP team uses a table with headers to provide pertinent data.

- Organizing or preparing the data from the evidence summary assists the team in conducting the next step of the process, evidence synthesis. This can be done with various visual and sorting tools.

- *Synthesis* is the process of creating greater meaning from the data provided by individual articles or reports.

- Synthesized evidence is used to generate best-evidence recommendations that answer the EBP question. Recommendations can be high-, reasonable-, reasonable-to-low-, or low-certainty.

OBJECTIVES

- 9.1 Differentiate between summary and synthesis (analyzing)
- 9.2 Develop a summary of the evidence (creating)
- 9.3 Develop a synthesis of the evidence (creating)
- 9.4 Select best-evidence recommendations (evaluating)

LEARNING ACTIVITIES

Before completion of the learning activities, you should do the following:

- Read Chapter 9
- Listen to this podcast: https://podcasts.apple.com/us/podcast/ep-6-johns-hopkins-nursing-center-for-nursing-inquiry/id1478145611?i=1000448670865
- Download the Best-Evidence Summary Tool (Appendix G1), Individual Evidence Summary Tool (Appendix G2), and Summary, Synthesis, & Best-Evidence Recommendations Tool (Appendix H)

Learning Activity 9.1

Using the following table, differentiate between summary and synthesis.

	SUMMARY	SYNTHESIS
Definition		
Purpose		
Content focus		
Depth of analysis		
Use in EBP		
Outcome		

Learning Activity 9.2

Using the evidence that you appraised in Learning Activity 8.4, summarize the evidence. Complete the Best-Evidence Summary Tool (Appendix G1; see Figure 9.1) and the Individual Evidence Summary Tool (Appendix G2; see Figure 9.2) as appropriate.

Best-Evidence Summary Tool — JOHNS HOPKINS NURSING

Purpose: This tool collates information from pre-appraised evidence identified in the best-evidence search and other data obtained from a targeted search. It brings all the data into a central document to help the EBP team with the next step of the EBP process, synthesis.

Section I: Pre-Appraised Evidence

Complete the data collection tool below for all included pre-appraised evidence.

Article Number	Author (organization), date, title	Type of pre-appraised evidence	Topic or Intervention	Population	Setting	Recommendations that answer the EBP question

Section II: Reports of Single Studies from the Targeted Evidence Search

Was there additional evidence identified in the targeted search?
- [ ] No → Skip to Section II of Appendix H
- [ ] Yes → Record information from evidence that provides strong or moderate support for decision-making in the table below.

Article number	Reviewer names	Author, date, and title	Type of evidence	Population, size, and setting	Intervention	Findings that help answer the EBP question	Measures used	Limitations	Moderate, or strong support for decision-making?

Complete Section II of Appendix H

FIGURE 9.1 Best-Evidence Summary Tool (Appendix G1).

Individual Evidence Summary Tool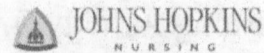

Purpose: This tool collates information from the literature gathered during the exhaustive evidence search. It brings all of the data into a central document to help the EBP team with the next step of the EBP process, synthesis.

Complete the data collection tool below for all included evidence from the exhaustive evidence search.

Article number	Reviewer names	Author, date, and title	Type of evidence	Population, size, and setting	Intervention	Findings that help answer the EBP question	Measures used	Limitations	Level of support for decision-making	Notes to the team

FIGURE 9.2 Individual Evidence Summary Tool (Appendix G2).

Learning Activity 9.3

Using the summary completed above, synthesize the evidence using section I of the Summary, Synthesis, & Best-Evidence Recommendations Tool (Appendix H; see Figure 9.3). Be sure to note the degree of support for decision-making for those recommendations. Also provide the summary of evidence from Appendix G1.

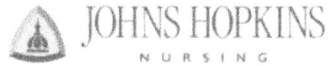

Summary, Synthesis, & Best-Evidence Recommendations Tool

Purpose: This tool guides the EBP team through the process of synthesizing the pertinent findings from the Best Evidence or Individual Evidence Summary (Appendix G1 or G2) to create an overall picture of the body of the evidence related to the EBP question. The team analyzes the data in each category of support for decision-making, as well as any additional organizational approaches that bring further insights.

Section I: Findings from the Individual Evidence Summary

Support for Decision-Making	Synthesized Findings with Article Number(s) *(This is not a simple restating of information from each individual evidence summary—see instructions)*
Strong Number of sources = _____	
Moderate Number of sources = _____	
Limited Number of sources = _____	

FIGURE 9.3 Summary, Synthesis, & Best-Evidence Recommendations Tool (Appendix H), section I.

Learning Activity 9.4

From the synthesis, develop the best-evidence recommendations, paying attention to the characteristics of the recommendations (see Figure 9.4). Write the recommendations as recommendations statements such as:

- There is high-certainty evidence supporting the use of warming blankets.
- There is reasonable-to-low certainty evidence to recommend that nurses take naps on the night shift.

Section II: Best-Evidence Recommendations

The recommendations below are based on:

☐ Pre-appraised evidence identified in a best evidence search → Record each recommendation in the corresponding evidence category in the table below based on the confidence/certainty listed in the clinical practice guidelines, evidence summary, or literature review with a systematic approach

☐ Evidence appraised by the EBP team from a targeted search to supplement the pre-appraised evidence (single studies with a formal study design) → Record any additional or altered recommendations to the pre-appraised evidence in the corresponding evidence category in table below. See instructions for more details.

☐ Evidence appraised by the EBP team from an exhaustive search (single studies, anecdotal evidence, and pre-appraised evidence that does not fully address the EBP question) → Record each recommendation in the table below based on the team's analysis and synthesis of information in Section I

Characteristics of the Recommendation(s)	Best-Evidence Recommendation(s)
High certainty recommendations (Robust, well-documented, consistent & persuasive, based mostly on evidence that provides strong support for decision-making)	
Reasonable certainty recommendations (Good, mostly compelling, consistent evidence, based mostly on evidence that provides moderate to strong support for decision-making)	
Characteristics of the Recommendation(s)	Recommendation(s) Lacking Adequate Evidence
Reasonable to low certainty recommendations (Good but conflicting evidence. Inconsistent results, based mostly on evidence that provides moderate support for decision making)	
Low certainty recommendations (Little to no evidence. Information is minimal, inconsistent and/or based mostly on evidence that provides limited support for decision-making)	

FIGURE 9.4 Summary, Synthesis, & Best-Evidence Recommendations Tool (Appendix H), section II.

CALL TO ACTION

1. Following the best-evidence search, complete the Best-Evidence Summary Tool (Appendix G1). Add any additional evidence gleaned from a targeted search.

2. Following the exhaustive search, complete the Individual Evidence Summary Tool (Appendix G2).

3. Once all of your included evidence has been summarized, synthesize the evidence using the Summary, Synthesis, & Best-Evidence Recommendations Tool (Appendix H, section I).

4. From this synthesis, develop best-evidence recommendations. Ensure the recommendations are aligned with the characteristics of the recommendations. Finish completing the Summary, Synthesis, & Best-Evidence Recommendations Tool (Appendix H, section II).

DISCUSSION QUESTIONS

1. Why is a thorough understanding of evidence crucial to the success of an EBP project, and what risks might an organization face if changes are implemented based on incomplete or poorly understood evidence?

2. What are the key components of a robust synthesis of evidence, and how can these components ensure the development of high-quality, best-evidence recommendations?

3. How does critical thinking contribute to the evaluation and synthesis of evidence, and in what ways can this skill enhance the overall effectiveness of an EBP project?

4. In what ways should patient and provider preferences be considered when translating evidence into organizational practice? Why is it essential to integrate these preferences into the decision-making process?

5. Reflect on a scenario where organizational change was implemented based on weak evidence. What lessons can be learned from such experiences, and how can they inform future EBP projects to ensure more reliable and impactful outcomes?

A CLOSER LOOK

The Best-Evidence Summary Tool summarizes the pre-appraised evidence found during a best-evidence search and any additional evidence found during a targeted search. By contrast, the Individual Evidence Summary Tool provides a summary of the single-study and anecdotal evidence found during an exhaustive search. The Summary, Synthesis, & Best-Evidence Recommendations Tool is used to synthesize the evidence and develop best-evidence recommendations. See Figures 9.5, 9.6, and 9.7.

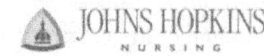

FIGURE 9.5 Best-Evidence Summary Tool (Appendix G1), annotated.

Individual Evidence Summary Tool

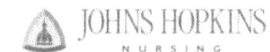

Purpose: This tool collates information from the literature. It brings all of the data into a central document to help the EBP team with the next step of the EBP process, synthesis.

Article number	Reviewer names	Author, date, and title	Type of evidence	Population, size, and setting	Intervention	Findings that help answer the EBP question	Measures used	Limitations	Level of support for decision-making	Notes to the team

Word bank for type of evidence:

No individual report will use a term from each column. Within each grouping, only select one term.

Reviews	Methodology	Design/Approach	Timing	Other
-Systematic with or without meta-analysis -Integrative -Rapid -Umbrella -Scoping -Critical -Literature	Quantitative Qualitative Mixed-Methods	Randomized Controlled Trial (RCT)	Prospective Retrospective	-Expert opinion -Book chapter experience

FIGURE 9.6 Individual Evidence Summary Tool (Appendix G2), annotated.

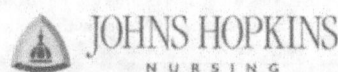

Summary, Synthesis, & Best-Evidence Recommendations Tool

Purpose: This tool guides the EBP team through the process of synthesizing [the] Evidence or Individual Evidence Summary (Appendix G1 or G2) to create an [evidence summary] related to the EBP question. The team analyzes the data in each category of [evidence and] any additional organizational approaches that bring further insights.

> Section 1 should only reflect evidence from the Individual Evidence Summary Tool (Appendix G2).

Section I: Findings from the Individual Evidence Summary	
Support for Decision-Making	**Synthesized Findings with Article Number(s)** *(This is not a simple restating of information from each individual evidence summary—see instructions)*
Strong Number of sources = _____	Synthesis identifies important takeaways from the collected evidence. The succinct synthesis statements should reflect a better understanding of the evidence to answer the EBP question.
Moderate Number of sources = _____	
Limited Number of sources = _____	Teams should include the article numbers used to generate the synthesized recommendations to make the original evidence easy to find.

Further Synthesis Based on Additional Organization and Analysis (OPTIONAL)
Sometimes teams may want to further categorize the findings according to identified themes, patterns, and subgroups. For example, when reviewing evidence around fall prevention, you may want to further categorize nurse-led, patient-led, and organization-led initiatives.

FIGURE 9.7 Summary, Synthesis, & Best-Evidence Recommendations Tool (Appendix H), annotated.

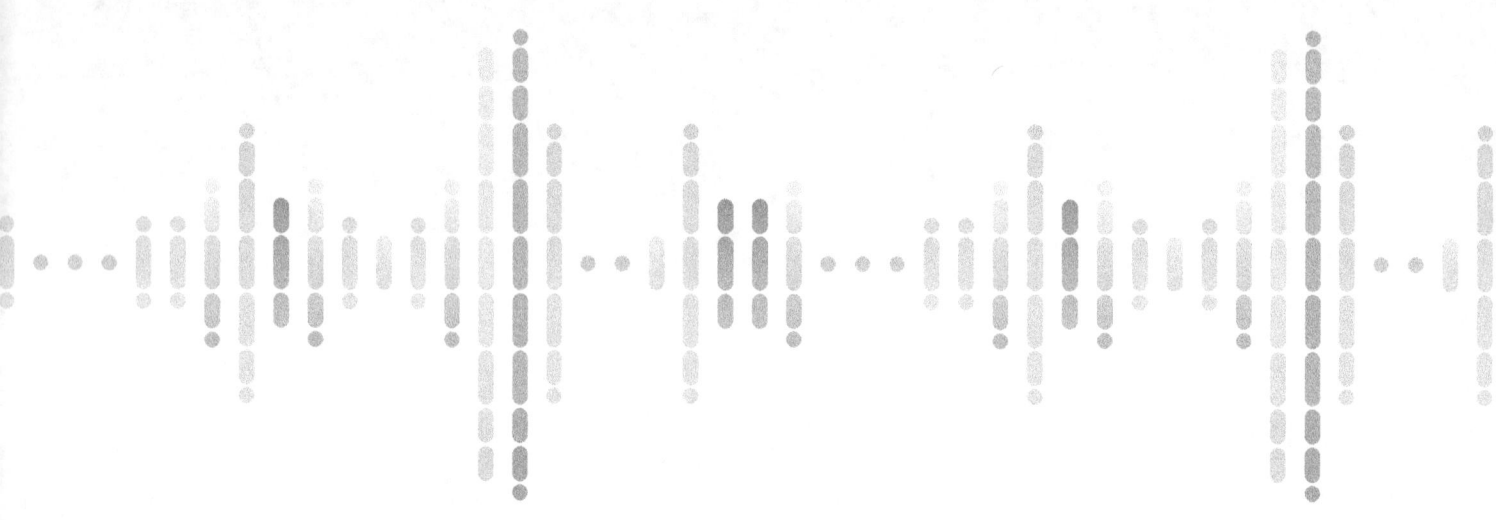

OVERVIEW

The final phase of the PET process is translation. This is the value-added step in an EBP project that could significantly impact clinical outcomes, patient safety and quality, leadership, and health policy (White et al., 2019). EBP teams may find evidence to support their current practice and continue without a change, or updates can occur in practice, process, or systems to influence targeted outcomes positively.

Through the translation process, the EBP team evaluates the best-evidence recommendations (identified in the evidence phase) for transferability to a desired practice setting. This step is followed by implementation, described in Chapter 11, with the potential for significant positive outcomes that can inspire and motivate the EBP team, revolutionizing healthcare practices and policies. The potential impact of the translation phase on healthcare practices and policies is significant, making the audience feel the importance and influence of their work in the EBP process.

10

TRANSLATION PHASE: TRANSLATION

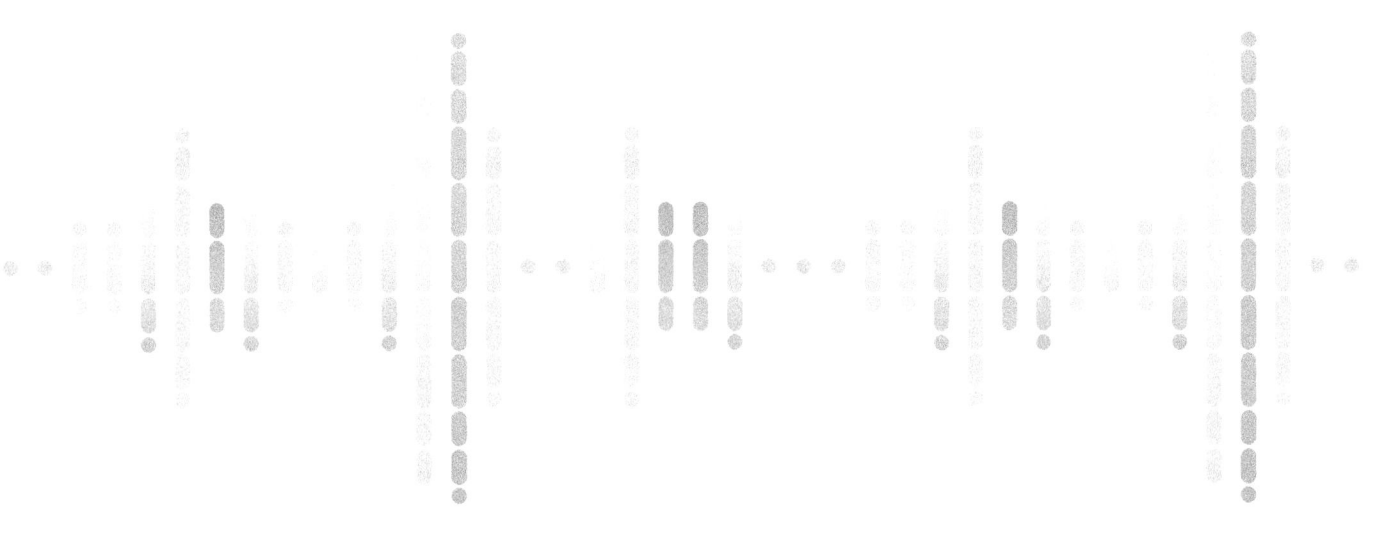

KEY POINTS

The translation phase contains six steps. This chapter gives an overview of Steps 11–12 to develop practice setting-specific recommendations from the evidence synthesis. Information in this chapter will assist the EBP team in completing the Translation Tool (Appendix I).

- *Translation* is the process of adapting or customizing evidence findings into the specific content into which they will be implemented.

- The EBP team needs to follow these steps to ensure that effective translation of each piece of evidence occurs:

    - Consider the certainty of each best-evidence recommendation.

    - Identify the potential negative impact on patient or staff safety.

    - *Fit* is accomplished by evaluating both the end-user and organizational characteristics.

- Assessing the practice environment's readiness to change is critical to determining the *feasibility* of evidence translation.

- Impacted groups are essential when establishing *acceptability* of the evidence.

- Tools exist that the EBP team can use to help inform organizational decision-making related to translation. The EBP team should make organization-specific recommendations and record them to ensure that all are clear so that implementation may proceed.

OBJECTIVES

- 10.1 Differentiate between fit, feasibility, and acceptability (analyzing)

- 10.2 Develop organization-specific recommendations (creating)

LEARNING ACTIVITIES

Before completion of the learning activities, you should do the following:

- Read Chapter 10
- Download the Translation Tool (Appendix I)

Learning Activity 10.1

Differentiate between fit, feasibility, and acceptability by completing the following table.

	FIT	FEASIBILITY	ACCEPTABILITY
Purpose			
Key Questions			

Learning Activity 10.2

Read the following case study excerpt.

After completing your exhaustive literature search, summarizing and synthesizing the evidence, and providing best-evidence recommendations, your EBP team needs to develop organization-specific recommendations. Recall that your organization-specific recommendations may slightly differ from the best-evidence recommendations, since the evidence may not accurately represent what is best for your specific hospital. Your organization-specific recommendations take into consideration your available resources, your strategic goals and priorities, and your staff preferences and experiences. Here is a snapshot of what is available on your unit:

- ***Available equipment:*** *Your unit has 25 semi-private rooms, shared by two patients. Each room is equipped with two televisions and two phones, one for each patient. There are no computers in the patient rooms, so clinicians use workstations on wheels to complete charting outside the patient room. Your unit does not own or use tablet devices. Your unit has discussed installing two whiteboards in each patient room, one for each patient, but this initiative has not rolled out.*

- ***Available staffing:*** *From a nursing perspective, your unit is adequately staffed. In addition to a team of bedside nurses, your unit employs a clinical nurse specialist, a nurse educator, and a team of unlicensed assistive personnel to support the bedside nurses. Your unit also has a core group of dedicated volunteers that visit with the patients and assist visitors. Despite adequate staffing, nursing and nursing support staff have high workloads. Often, staff do not have the bandwidth to add additional tasks to their already demanding workloads.*

- ***Available funding:*** *Your hospital has limited funding to spend on new initiatives.*

The case study excerpt provides some insights about fit, feasibility, and acceptability around the best-evidence recommendations. Using the following table, in concise statements develop organization-specific recommendations that address the EBP question.

BEST-EVIDENCE RECOMMENDATION	ORGANIZATION-SPECIFIC RECOMMENDATION

CALL TO ACTION

Determine the risk, fit, feasibility, and acceptability of the best-evidence recommendations for translation into your organization. Using that assessment, develop organization-specific recommendations. Complete the Translation Tool (Appendix I; see Figure 10.1).

Translation Tool

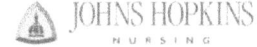

Purpose: This tool guides the EBP team through analyzing the best-evidence recommendations for translation into the team's specific setting. The translation process considers the certainty, risk, feasibility, fit, and acceptability of the best-evidence recommendations. The team uses both critical thinking and clinical reasoning to generate site-specific recommendations.

Refer to the recommendations developed on Appendix H. Consider the certainty of *each* best-evidence recommendation, as well as the fit, feasibility, acceptability, and risk to develop organization-specific recommendations.

Certainty	Risk	Fit	Feasibility	Acceptability
• Do the recommendations have high or reasonable certainty? (Recommendations with reasonable to low and low certainty do not provide adequate support to change current practice, *see instructions below*)	• What is the potential negative impact on patient or staff safety? (Interventions with higher risk require higher certainty evidence to put into practice.)	• How well does the change align with existing practices? • Values? • Norms? • Goals? • Skills?	• Is the change doable and are barriers realistic to overcome? • Is the practice environment ready for change? • Are necessary materials or human resources available? • Can the change be successfully implemented?	• Do impacted groups find the change agreeable? • Does leadership support the change and trust it is reasonable? • Does the change align with organizational priorities?

In concise statements, record the organization-specific recommendations below that address the EBP question.

FIGURE 10.1 Translation Tool (Appendix I).

DISCUSSION QUESTIONS

1. What organizational considerations should be evaluated when deciding whether to implement a practice change based on evidence? How can factors like safety risk, fit, feasibility, and acceptability impact the success of the translation process?

2. Why is assessing organizational readiness critical before translating evidence into practice? What challenges might arise if this step is overlooked or insufficiently conducted?

3. What steps can an EBP team take to ensure that an intervention not only fits well within the organization but also is feasible and acceptable to impacted groups? Why are these considerations important for sustaining the practice change?

4. How can an EBP project benefit from using a structured framework to guide the translation process? What are some potential risks if a project moves forward without such a framework?

A CLOSER LOOK

The Translation Tool (Appendix I)

This tool (see Figure 10.2) guides the team in developing organization-specific recommendations from the best-evidence recommendations. Teams consider risk, fit, feasibility, and acceptability of recommendations within their setting.

Translation Tool

JOHNS HOPKINS NURSING

Purpose: This tool guides the EBP team through the translation process considers the certainty, risk, and clinical reasoning to generate site-specific recommendations. The team uses both critical thinking and clinical reasoning to generate site-specific recommendations.

> Determine the risk, feasibility, fit, and acceptability for each high and reasonable certainty recommendation identified in section II of the Summary, Synthesis, & Best-Evidence Recommendations Tool (Appendix H).

Refer to the recommendations developed on Appendix H, and consider the certainty of the recommendation, as well as the fit, feasibility, acceptability, and risk to develop organization-specific recommendations.

Certainty	Risk	Fit	Feasibility	Acceptability
• Do the recommendations have high or reasonable certainty? (Recommendations with reasonable to low and low certainty do not provide adequate support to change current practice, *see instructions below*)	• What is the potential negative impact on patient or staff safety? (Interventions with higher risk require higher certainty evidence to put into practice.)	• How well does the change align with existing practices? • Values? • Norms? • Goals? • Skills?	• Is the change doable and are barriers realistic to overcome? • Is the practice environment ready for change? • Are necessary materials or human resources available? • Can the change be successfully implemented?	• Do impacted groups find the change agreeable? • Does leadership support the change and trust it is reasonable? • Does the change align with organizational priorities?

In concise statements, record the organization-specific recommendations below that address the EBP question.

> Recommendations should reflect the evaluation of certainty, risk, fit, feasibility, and acceptability pertinent to the organization.

> Note: A recommendation may be to do nothing or to de-implement an existing practice.

FIGURE 10.2 Translation Tool (Appendix I), annotated.

REFERENCE

White, K. M., Dudley-Brown, S., & Terhaar, M. (2019). *Translation of evidence into nursing and healthcare* (3rd ed.). Springer.

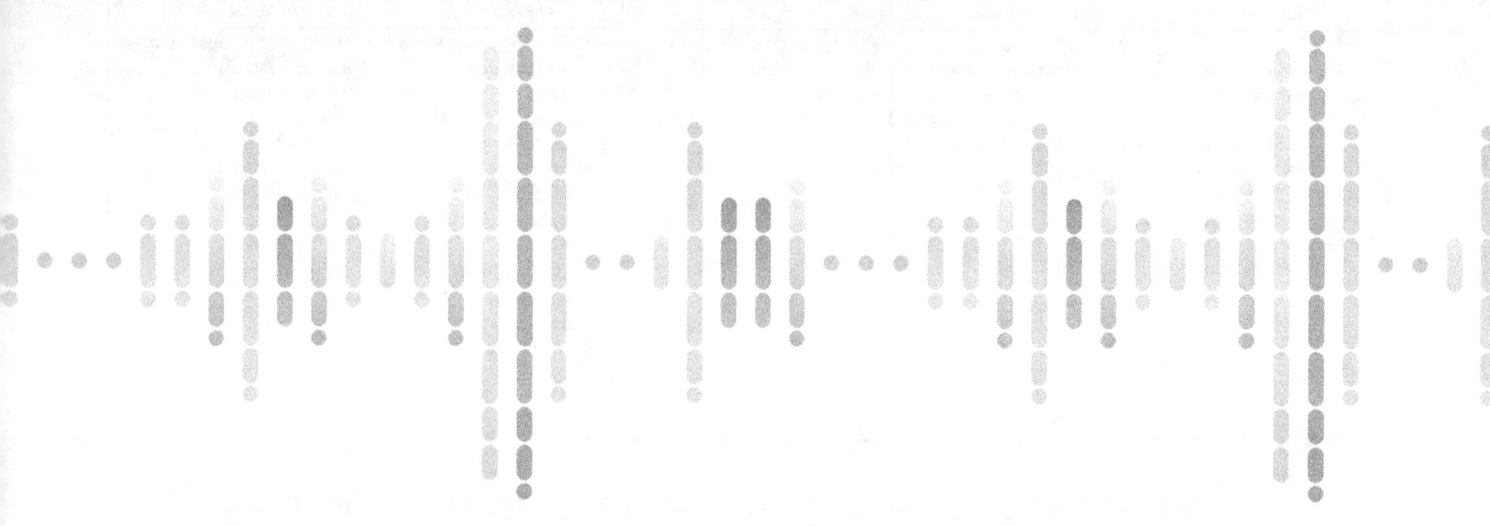

OVERVIEW

After the EBP team has determined if a practice change is indicated and translated the best evidence to their practice setting, the next task is to implement the change. Implementation is one of the final steps of the EBP process and is essential to bring the best evidence to the bedside. To ensure not only success but also sustainability, the EBP team should be deliberate in the planning and execution of their intervention or innovation (White et al., 2019). Three keys to successful implementation are selecting and using project management tool(s), an implementation framework or model with a timeline, and a sustainability plan.

11

TRANSLATION PHASE: IMPLEMENTATION

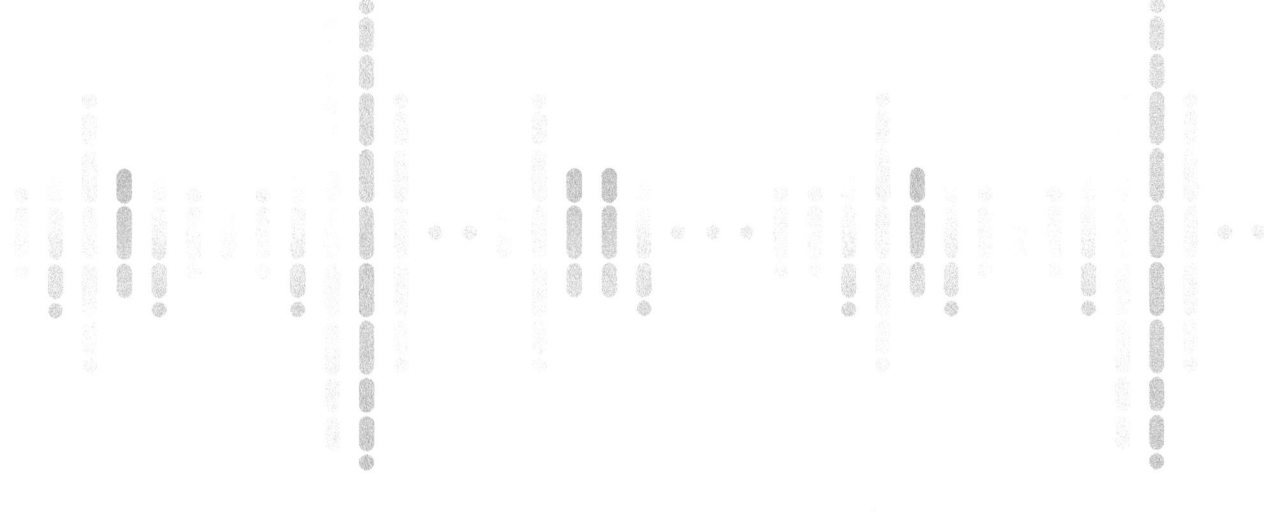

KEY POINTS

The translation phase contains six steps. This chapter provides an overview of the final steps (13–16) to implement any changes identified in Step 12. Information in this chapter will assist the EBP team in completing the JHEBP Implementation and Action Planning (A3) Tool (Appendix J).

- Selecting the correct project management tools is crucial for successful EBP implementation.

- The *A3 tool* is a project plan that consolidates the entire project implementation into one tool.

- A detailed project timeline can be incorporated into the project's A3.

- A *Gantt chart* is a high-level visual representation where a Work Breakdown Structure (WBS) tool is more granular in identifying specific tasks and when they need to be completed.

- Identifying an implementation framework to help guide your project implementation can enhance the efficiency, effectiveness, and sustainability of your implementation.

- The *TRIP model* is an implementation framework that works well with the JHEBP model.

- A sustainability plan is imperative to ensure that project changes outlast the closure of the project.

OBJECTIVES

- 11.1 Develop SMART goals to guide implementation (creating)

- 11.2 Identify appropriate metrics for a given project (understanding)

- 11.3 Complete a Work Breakdown Structure outlining the implementation plan (understanding)

LEARNING ACTIVITIES

Before completion of the learning activities, you should do the following:

- Read Chapter 11
- Download the Implementation and Action Planning (A3) Tool (Appendix J; Hopkins.org/tools)

Learning Activity 11.1

Read the following case study excerpt.

Due to the limited funding and technology on your unit, your unit has decided to implement a low-tech modality to engage patients and families in the fall prevention care plan. Your unit is going to install laminated fall prevention posters at each bedside. The posters will display a list of fall risk factors (e.g., history of falls, medication side effects, ambulatory aid, walking ability, IV pole or equipment, unsteady gait, and forgetting or choosing not to call for help) and a list of preventative measures (e.g., use assistance when walking, use ambulatory aids, frequent toileting, bed alarms, etc.). The poster will be hung in a location that is easy to access and visualize.

A healthcare worker or volunteer will sit with the patient and family within 48 hours of admission to determine which risk factors apply to the patient and which preventative measures are most suitable to the patient. Bedside nurses, unlicensed assistive personnel, and volunteers will all be trained in how to use the fall prevention posters. The bedside nurse will be responsible for either completing the fall prevention poster with the patient and family or delegating the task to an unlicensed assistive personnel or volunteer. This intervention is in addition to your current patient education plan.

If the intervention results in an improvement after six months of implementation, your unit would like to install whiteboards at each bedside to use instead of the laminated posters.

Using the recommendations identified in Chapter 10, Learning Activity 10.2, identify two metrics appropriate for measuring the impact of the implementation.

1. _____

2. _____

Learning Activity 11.2

Using the excerpt above and the responses for Learning Activity 11.1, write three SMART goals related to implementing the identified organization-specific recommendations.

1. _____

2. _____

3. _____

Learning Activity 11.3

Continuing with the case study excerpt, identify three high-level deliverables important to implementing the recommendations and ensuring success. Add them to the first column in the following table.

HIGH-LEVEL DELIVERABLE	ASSOCIATED TASKS AND SUB-TASKS	START DATE	END DATE	RESPONSIBLE PARTY	RESOURCES NEEDED

CALL TO ACTION

As a team, identify an implementation framework that works with your project. Complete the Implementation and Action Planning (A3) Tool (Appendix J; see Figure 11.1).

Problem/Evidence (summary of problem, synthesis of evidence)	Implementation (Educate, Execute)
Goal	
SMART Goal aligned with Strategic Priority:	
Key Accomplishments using Translation Framework:	

Timeline/Milestones (Gantt)	People (Engage)
	Project Leader: Working Group: Collaborating Groups: Impacted Groups: Sponsor:

Metrics Progress (Evaluate)

Risk and Risk Mitigation Strategy		
Risk	Risk Mitigation Strategy	Status

Work Breakdown Structure (refer to the Timeline/Milestones section of A3 and provide details for each phase of the implementation framework)							
Due Date	Task	Dependencies	Accountable Person(s)	Status	Planned Completion	Actual Completion	Resource

Sustainability Plan (Endure)							
What are the potential barriers to project sustainability?	What are some mitigation strategies for the potential obstacles?	What additional resources may be needed to support the project?	What additional training may be required?	What responsibilities need to be assigned?	To whom will these responsibilities be assigned?	Are there any additional metrics/outcomes that need to be collected/measured?	How frequently will you monitor and review your outcomes?

FIGURE 11.1 Implementation and Action Planning (A3) Tool (Appendix J).

Use this tool to guide the implementation of the organization-specific recommendations. Remember to consider the impacted parties throughout this process. Additionally, you may need to build a team specific to implementation. Implement the organization-specific recommendations.

DISCUSSION QUESTIONS

1. How does the TRIP model facilitate the translation of evidence-based recommendations into practice, and what are the key components of this implementation framework?
2. What role do goal setting and timeline creation play in the success of an EBP project's implementation phase, and how can these elements be adapted when using other implementation frameworks?
3. What strategies can an EBP team employ to identify and mitigate barriers to implementation, and why is it important to address these challenges early in the process?

4. Why is a sustainability plan essential for EBP projects, and what factors should be considered to ensure that practice changes are maintained beyond project completion?

5. How can the use of communication strategies both within the EBP team and across the organization enhance the effectiveness of the implementation and contribute to long-term sustainability of the practice change?

A CLOSER LOOK

The Implementation and Action Planning (A3) Tool (Appendix J)

This tool (see Figure 11.2) summarizes the project and provides a standardized process for teams, consolidating an entire project into one document to facilitate communication on progress to teammates, peers, and leadership. It can be modified to meet the team's needs.

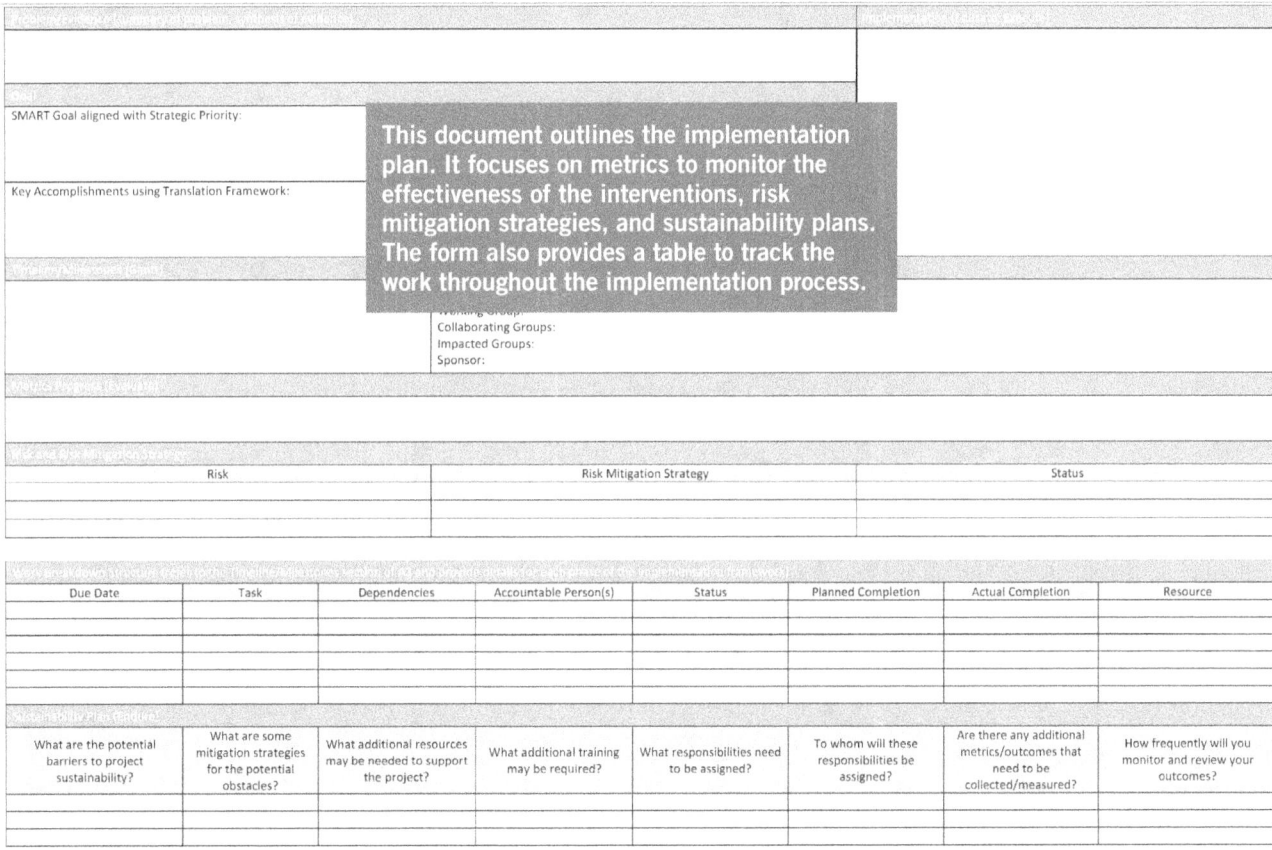

FIGURE 11.2 Implementation and Action Planning (A3) Tool (Appendix J), annotated.

REFERENCE

White, K. M., Dudley-Brown, S., & Terhaar, M. (2019). *Translation of evidence into nursing and healthcare* (3rd ed.). Springer.

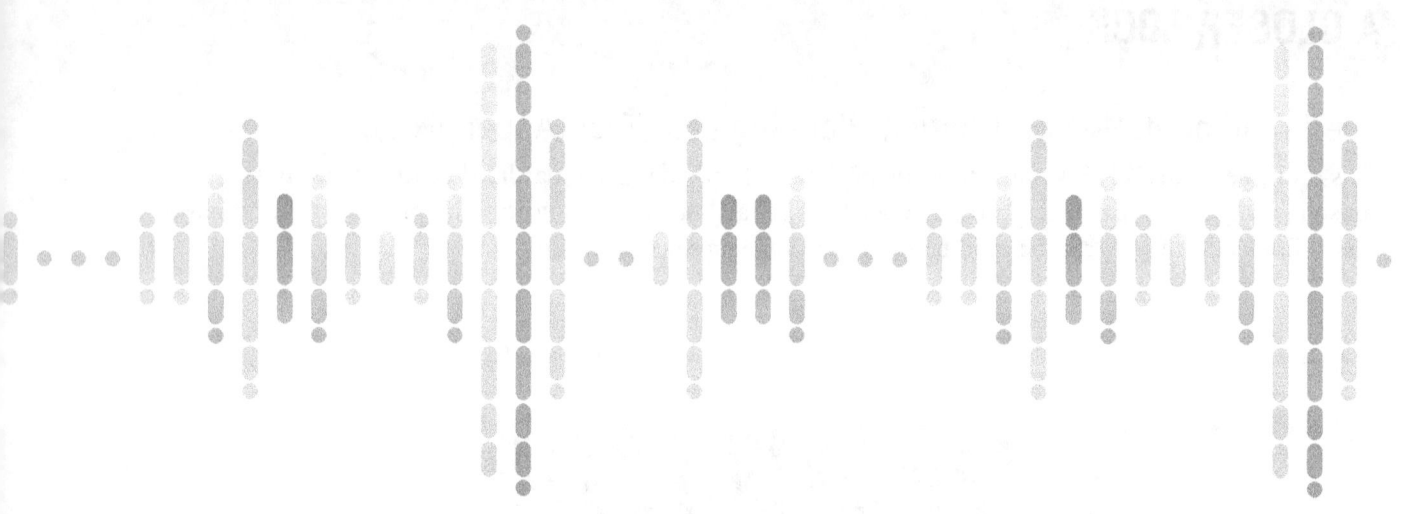

OVERVIEW

Dissemination of EBP projects can take various forms and is an essential step in the EBP process. As members of the healthcare community, the EBP team can improve knowledge accessibility, enhance the state of science on a given topic, and catalyze change.

The importance of dissemination cannot be discounted and has even been included in healthcare providers' codes of ethics, including the American Nurses Association (ANA) and the American Medical Association (AMA). These documents call for the advancement of the profession through various scientific approaches, including research development, evaluation, prompt dissemination, and application to practice (AMA, 2016; ANA, 2015).

Clinically practicing healthcare providers completing an EBP project are in the unique position to provide firsthand knowledge of patient care coupled with best-practice evidence and realistic recommendations. Dissemination is a tool to advocate for patients, staff, and populations and is an opportunity for the EBP team to translate evidence into clinical practice and promote science and healthcare professions.

12

ONGOING CONSIDERATIONS: COMMUNICATION AND DISSEMINATION

KEY POINTS

Dissemination can occur throughout the EBP project. Resources to facilitate the process include the Impacted Groups Analysis and Communication Resource and the Reporting Guidelines for EBP Projects at Hopkins.org/resources.

- There are five components of an effective dissemination plan, including purpose, message, audience, timing, and method.

- *Internal dissemination* refers to sharing information with groups within a team's organization.

- Communication strategies should be tailored for unit-, departmental-, and organization-level groups. Executive summaries can be an effective communication strategy for executive leadership.

- *External dissemination* refers to sharing information outside a team's organization.

- Venues for external dissemination include conferences, peer-reviewed journals, and social media.

- Communication and dissemination are essential components of an EBP project. Not only are they mandates by healthcare associations, such as the ANA, but they are also essential for improving care for patients and advancing the science of healthcare.

OBJECTIVES

- 12.1 Identify the key components of a dissemination plan (understanding)

- 12.2 Consider the impacted groups identified previously, and craft messages according to the audience (Impacted Groups Analysis and Communication Resource) (creating)

- 12.3 Identify important components of an executive summary (understanding)

LEARNING ACTIVITIES

Before completion of the learning activities, you should do the following:

- Read Chapter 12
- Listen to this podcast: https://podcasts.apple.com/us/podcast/ep-37-i-was-published-in-a-scholarly-journal-you/id1478145611?i=1000575529262
- Review the Impacted Groups Analysis and Communication Resource and the Reporting Guidelines for EBP Projects (Hopkins.org/resources)

Learning Activity 12.1

Identify the key components of a dissemination plan by filling in the following blanks.

1. _____: will drive all other factors; examples may be to raise awareness, educate, or share results.

2. _____: should be clear, targeted, and repeated several times; a call to action.

3. _____: messaging should be adjusted according to the recipients, their needs, and their background.

4. _____: consider when messages should be conveyed; often requires repeated messaging.

5. _____: approach to messaging should match the audience; a variety of channels should be used.

Learning Activity 12.2

Considering the recommendations and plan, craft key messages and align with methods for the frontline nurses. Fill them out in the Communication Planning section of the Impacted Groups Analysis and Communication Resource (see Figure 12.1).

Communication Planning			
Refer to this section to guide your communications to the impacted groups throughout and after completing the EBP project.			
What is the purpose of the dissemination of the EBP project findings? (check all that apply) ☐ Raise awareness ☐ Change practice ☐ Inform impacted groups ☐ Promote action ☐ Engage impacted groups ☐ Other:_____ ☐ Change policy			
What are the 3 most important messages?			
Align key message(s) and methods with the audience:			
Audience	Key Messages	Method	Timing
Interdisciplinary groups			
Organizational leadership			
Frontline nurses			
Departmental leadership			
External community			
Other			

FIGURE 12.1 Impacted Groups Analysis and Communication Resource.

Learning Activity 12.3

Using the word bank provided, develop a logical outline for an executive summary. Create your outline in the left column below.

	Project outcomes
	Sustainability plan
	Steps of the Work Breakdown Structure (WBS)
	Organizational implications
	Evidence appraisal
	Why change is needed
	Literature review
	Current state of the problem
	Overview of the project (align with strategic priorities)
	Evaluation metrics
	List of evidence reviewed
	PRISMA diagram
	Implementation process
	Schedule of outcome measurement

> **CALL TO ACTION**
>
> If you have reached this point, hopefully, you have successfully implemented your project. If so, congratulations! It is now time to communicate and disseminate:
>
> - Create a communication plan for your impacted parties using the Impacted Groups Analysis and Communication Resource.
> - Craft an executive summary for organizational leadership.
> - Submit your project as an abstract for a podium or poster presentation.
> - Finally, use the Reporting Guidelines for EBP Projects to submit for publication.

DISCUSSION QUESTIONS

1. What are the various forms of dissemination available for EBP projects, and how can the choice of dissemination method impact the reach and influence of the project's findings?
2. Why is dissemination considered an ethical responsibility for healthcare providers, and how is this reflected in professional codes of ethics such as those from the ANA and AMA?
3. How can effective dissemination of EBP projects contribute to advancing the healthcare profession and improving patient care? What role does accessibility to knowledge play in this process?
4. In what ways does the unique perspective of clinically practicing healthcare providers enhance the value of disseminated EBP findings, particularly when it comes to realistic recommendations and best practices?
5. How can EBP teams use dissemination as a tool to advocate for specific patient populations or healthcare improvements? What considerations should be made to ensure that the advocacy efforts are both impactful and evidence-based?

A CLOSER LOOK

The Impacted Groups Analysis and Communication Resource

This resource (see Figure 12.2) prompts teams to identify potential impacted groups and plan communication. It is not meant to be completed only at one time point but referenced throughout the project.

Impacted Groups Analysis

Identify the key impacted groups:

- ☐ Manager or direct supervisor
- ☐ Finance department
- ☐ Vendors
- ☐ Patients and/or families; patient and family advisory committee
- ☐ Professional organizations
- ☐ Committees
- ☐ Organizational leaders
- ☐ Interdisciplinary colleagues (e.g., physicians, nutritionists, respiratory therapists, or OT/PT)
- ☐ Administrators
- ☐ Other units or departments
- ☐ Others: _____

Impacted Groups Analysis Matrix: (Adapted from http://www.tools4dev.org/)

Impacted Individual/Group Name and Title:	Role: (select all that apply) Responsibility, Approval, Consult, Inform	Impact Level: How much does the project impact them? (minor, moderate, significant)	Influence Level: How much influence do they have over the project? (minor, moderate, significant)	What matters most to the indiviual or group?	How could they contribute to the project?	How could they impede the project?	Strategy(s) for engaging them:
One individual or group may have more than one role.		*The team should identify people with a vested interest, role, and/or responsibility in the project. For example, approval of a policy may fall to unit leaders, whereas clinicians may provide consultation on feasibility.*			*Spending time identifying the potential contributions and impediments of each individual or group helps the team strategize for a successful implementation.*		

Communication Planning

Refer to this section to guide your communications t[o...]

The reporting section may be helpful at any stage of the process but is particularly useful when the team is ready to disseminate their findings. The three most important messages may only be evident once recommendations are determined. However, teams can use this structure to develop and tailor any type of communication.

What is the purpose of the dissemination of the EBP p[roject]?

- ☐ Raise awareness
- ☐ Promote action
- ☐ Change policy
- ☐ Change p[ractice]
- ☐ Engage i[n...]

What are the 3 most important messages?

Teams should consider multiple modalities for communicating the key messages. Think of delivering them multiple times and in multiple ways.

Align key message(s) and methods with the audience:

Audience	Key Messages	Timing
Interdisciplinary groups		
Organizational leadership		
Frontline nurses		
Departmental leadership		
External community		
Other		

Align the key message with the audience. People are interested in what change means to them and how they may be affected. Refer back to the matrix to see what each impacted individual values. Carefully tailoring the message to the audience ensures their concerns are met.

FIGURE 12.2 Impacted Groups Analysis and Communication Resource, annotated.

REFERENCES

American Medical Association. (2016). *AMA principles of medical ethics.* https://www.ama-assn.org/delivering-care/ama-principles-medical-ethics

American Nurses Association. (2015). *Code of ethics for nurses with interpretive statements.* https://www.nursingworld.org/practice-policy/nursing-excellence/ethics/code-of-ethics-for-nurses/coe-view-only/

www.ingramcontent.com/pod-product-compliance
Lightning Source LLC
Chambersburg PA
CBHW082213300426

44117CB00016B/2789